Praises for Bragg Health[...]
and the Bragg Healthy Heart Book

These are just a few of the thousands of testimonials we receive yearly, praising The Bragg Health Books for the Super Health and rejuvenation benefits they reap – physically, mentally and spiritually. We also look forward to hearing from you soon.

When I was a young gymnastics coach at Stanford University, Paul Bragg's words and example inspired me to live a healthy lifestyle. I was 23 then; now over 63, and my own health and fitness serves as a living testimonial to Bragg's wisdom, carried on by Patricia, his dedicated health crusading daughter. I Thank You Both!
– Dan Millman, Author of "Way of the Peaceful Warrior"
• *www.danmillman.com*

Paul Bragg saved my life at age 15 when I attended the Bragg Health Crusade in Oakland, California. I went from sickness to total health. I thank Bragg Healthy Lifestyle for my long life. I now love sharing health with everyone!
– Jack LaLanne, Bragg follower since 15 • *www.jacklalanne.com*

Thank you Paul and Patricia Bragg for my simple, easy to follow Bragg Healthy Lifestyle. You make my days healthy!
– Clint Eastwood, Academy Award Winning Film Producer, Director, Actor and Bragg follower for over 50 years

In Medical School I read Dr. Bragg's Health Books. They changed my way of thinking and the path of my life. I founded Omega Institute.
– Stephan Rechtschaffen, M.D. • *www.eomega.org*

Thanks to Paul Bragg and Bragg Books, my years of asthma were cured in one month with Bragg Healthy Lifestyle Living!
– Paul Wenner, Gardenburger Creator • *www.gardenburger.com*

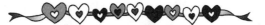

A fast with distilled or purified water can help you heal with greater speed; cleanse your liver, kidneys and colon; purify your blood; help you lose excess weight and bloating; flush out toxins; clear the eyes, tongue, and cleanse the breath. I thank Bragg Health Books for my conversion to the healthy way.
– James F. Balch, M.D., Co-Author, *Prescription for Nutritional Healing*

a

Praises for Bragg Healthy Lifestyle and the Bragg Healthy Heart Book

As a youth I had a learning disability and was told I would never read, write or communicate normally. At the age of 14 I dropped out of school and at 17 ended up in Hawaii surfing. My road to recovery led me to Paul Bragg who changed my life by giving me one simple affirmation to repeat: "I am a genius and I apply my wisdom." Bragg inspired me to live a healthy lifestyle and go back to school and get my education and from there miracles happened. I've authored 54 training programs and 14 books and love to health crusade around the world.
– Dr. John Demartini, Dynamic Crusader in "The Secret"
• *www.drdemartini.com*

Thanks to the Bragg Health Books, they were our introduction to healthy living. We are very grateful to you and your father. – Marilyn Diamond, Co-Author "Fit For Life"

Paul Bragg inspired me many years ago with the "Miracle of Fasting" and with his philosophy on health. His daughter Patricia is a testament to the ageless value of living the Bragg Healthy Lifestyle. – Jay Robb, author of *The Fruit Flush*

I have known Bragg Books over 30 years. They are a blessing to me and my family and to all who read them to help make this a healthier world. – Pastor Mike MacIntosh, Horizon Christian Fellowship, San Diego, CA • *horizonsd.org*

I've been reading Bragg Books since high school. I'm thankful for the healthy lifestyle and admire their health crusading to make this a healthier world!
– Steve Jobs, Creator & CEO – Apple Computer/iPods

Thanks to Bragg *Miracle of Fasting* and *Healthy Lifestyle* books, we are healthy, fit and singing better and staying younger than ever!
– The Beach Boys • *www.beachboysfanclub.com*

I am following the Bragg Healthy Lifestyle which I heard of through a friend. Your books are motivators and have blessed my health and life and are making perfect gifts for my family and friends. – Delphine, Singapore

b

Praises for Bragg Healthy Lifestyle and the Bragg Healthy Heart Book

I love the Bragg Books, especially *The Miracle of Fasting*. They are so popular and loved in Russia and the Ukraine. I give thanks for my health and my super energy. I won the famous Honolulu Marathon with the all-time women's record!
– Lyubov Morgunova, Champion Runner, Moscow, Russia

Thank you Patricia for our first meeting in London in 1968. When I was feeling my years, you gave me your *Miracle of Fasting* Book – it got me exercising – doing brisk walking and eating more wisely. You were a blessing God-sent and just when I needed to get more healthily recharged for crusading.
– Reverend Billy Graham

Your dad, Dr. Paul Bragg IS the FATHER of the natural health industry and the entire natural health movement. Everything that has been done in natural health and physical culture since has been based on the pioneering vision and principles articulated by Dr. Bragg. He gave us all our health direction!
– Dr. William Wong • *www.drwong.us*

In 1975 I was diagnosed with coronary heart disease. I followed the Free Bragg Exercise Classes and Health Lectures at Fort DeRussy lawn, Waikiki Beach, 6 days a week. 31 years have passed and I am going strong and healthy. Now 84 years young thanks to The Bragg Healthy Lifestyle. In 1932 my father had severe hip arthritis and was hardly able to walk. He followed the Bragg Healthy Lifestyle, also had the Bragg Vinegar Drink and he cured his arthritis.
– Helen Risk, RN, Hawaii

You've recharged me with hope, encouragement and love which poured from your words. I'm now able to fast and no more cigarettes and coffee for me, you've certainly improved my life!
– Marie Furia, New Jersey

Happiness is when . . . what you think, what you say, how you live, and what you do are in peaceful harmony. – Mahatma Gandhi

c

Praises for Bragg Healthy Lifestyle and the Bragg Healthy Heart Book

The Bragg Healthy Lifestyle with Fasting has changed my life! I lost weight and my energy levels went through the roof. I look forward to "Fasting" days. I think better and I am a better husband and father. Thank you Patricia, this has been a great blessing in my life. Also, thank you for your sharing the Bragg Healthy Lifestyle at our "AOL" Conference.
– Byron H. Elton, VP Entertainment, Time Warner AOL

I give thanks to Health Crusaders Paul Bragg and daughter Patricia for their dedicated years of service spreading health as our Lord wants us healthy! It's made a great difference in my life and millions worldwide. – Pat Robertson, Host CBN "700" Club

Paul C. Bragg and daughter Patricia were my early guiding inspiration to my health education and career.
– Jeffery Bland, Ph.D., Famous Food Scientist

I'd like to thank you for teaching me how to take control of my health! I have lost 55 pounds. I feel "Great"! Bragg books have showed me vitality, happiness and being close to Mother Nature. You are real "Crusaders of Health". – Leonard Amato

Dear Friends – you can not know how greatly you have already impacted my life and many of my friends and family! We love your Bragg Health Books, teachings and products, and we are now living healthier, happier lives. Thank You!
– Winnie Brown, Arizona

For over 35 years I have followed The Bragg Healthy Lifestyle. Bragg teaches you how to take control of your health and build a healthy, happy, long lasting, fulfilled future.
– Mark Victor Hansen, Co-Producer, "Chicken Soup for The Soul"

I am a big fan of Paul Bragg. I fast and use the Bragg Aminos daily on my food. I even take it with me when I travel for my seminars, I wouldn't be without it! The world and I are blessed with the health teachings of Paul and Patricia Bragg!
– Anthony "Tony" Robbins • *www.anthonyrobbins.com*

d

Praises for Bragg Healthy Lifestyle and the Bragg Healthy Heart Book

It was in Hawaii when I began to realize that while lifestyle choices can not only be a major negative to health and well-being, but lifestyle can be a winning asset to wellness! My discovery on fitness and health began shortly after I arrived in Hawaii at age 19 when I discovered Paul Bragg, the great health and fitness pioneer teaching a free exercise class 6 days a week at Waikiki Beach.
– Kathy Smith, Hollywood, CA • *www.kathysmith.com*

Our lives have completely turned around! Our family is feeling so very healthy and good, we must tell you about it.
– Gene & Joan Zollner, Parents of 11, Washington

I was diagnosed with diabetes and had high sugar levels. Following Bragg for 6 months, I was insulin free. I am healthier now than I have been for the last 15 years. My wife, three children and I are now healthy vegetarians living the Bragg Healthy Lifestyle. Results have been amazing. We thank You.
– Dennis Urbans, Australia

Daily we get letters at our Santa Barbara headquarters. We would love to hear from you on any blessings, healings and impact on your life you experienced after following The Bragg Healthy Lifestyle. It's all within your grasp to be in top health! By following this book, you can reap Super Health and a happy, long, vital life! It's never too late to begin – see (page 95) the study they did with people in their 80's and 90's and the amazing results that were obtained! You can receive miracles with nutrition, exercise and some fasting! Start now!

Daily our prayers & love go out to you, your heart, mind & soul.

Patricia and Paul C. Bragg

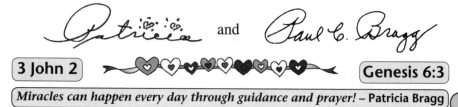

Miracles can happen every day through guidance and prayer! – Patricia Bragg

e

BRAGG PHOTO GALLERY

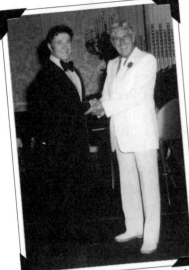

Thanks for The Bragg Healthy Lifestyle that you shared with me and are sharing with millions of others world-wide.

– John Gray, Ph.D., Author

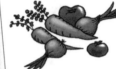

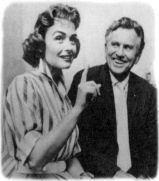

Actress Donna Reed saying "Health First" with Paul Bragg

Paul Bragg, Creator of Health Food Stores, with his prize student Jack LaLanne, who thanks Bragg for saving his life at 15.

PAUL C. BRAGG, ND, PhD.

Life Extension Specialist and Originator of Health Food Stores

In Medical School I read Dr. Bragg's Health Books, they changed my way of thinking & the path of my life. I founded Omega Institute. – Stephan Rechtschaffen, M.D. www.eomega.org • famous since 1977

Thanks to Paul Bragg & Daughter Patricia for my easy-to-follow Health Program. You make my days healthy. – Clint Eastwood Bragg Follower over 55 years

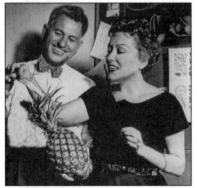

Paul Bragg with Actress Gloria Swanson who became a Bragg devotee when 18. She often health crusaded with Bragg.

I'd like to thank you for teaching me how to take control of my health! I lost 55 pounds and I feel "great"! Bragg books have showed me vitality, happiness and being close to Mother Nature. You both are real "Crusaders for Health for the World". Thanks. – Leonard Amato

I lost 102 lbs. with Bragg Apple Cider Vinegar and The Bragg Healthy Lifestyle and have kept it off for over 15 years, staying away from white flour, sugar and other processed foods. – Dee McCaffrey, Chemist & Diet Counselor, Tempe, AZ

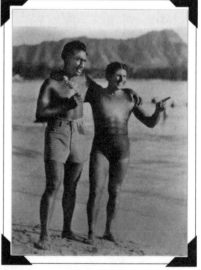

Paul Bragg with Duke Kahanamoku, the Olympic swimmer who taught Paul how to surf. His beautiful wife Nadine was Patricia's godmother.

f

PHOTO GALLERY

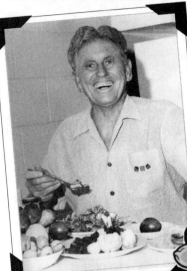

The Bragg Healthy Lifestyle teaches us all to be healthy, fit and ageless.
– Mark Victor Hansen, Co-Producer "Chicken Soup for the Soul" Series

PAUL BRAGG STAYING HEALTHY & FIT!

Paul Bragg in Tahiti (1925) gathering tropical papaya fruit.

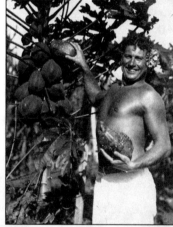

Paul Bragg owes his powerful body and superb health to living exclusively on live, vital, healthy, organic rich foods.

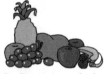

Paul C. Bragg and daughter Patricia were my early guiding inspiration to my health education and health career.
– Jeffery Bland, Ph.D., Famous Food Scientist

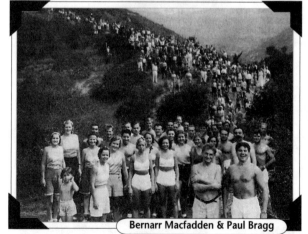

Bernarr Macfadden & Paul Bragg

A thousand happy Bragg Health Students enjoy hiking, exercise and fresh air on the trail to Mount Hollywood (above Griffith Observatory) in beautiful California, summer of 1932.

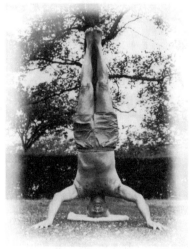

Paul C. Bragg at Regent's Park, London

PHOTO GALLERY

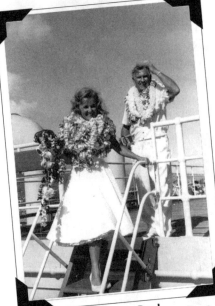

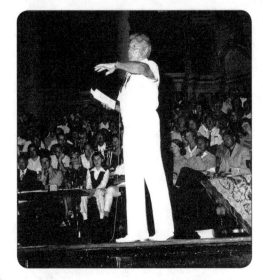

PAUL & PATRICIA BRAGG
HEALTH CRUSADING

Patricia and father, Paul on world trip in 1950's, during stop in Tahiti.

During the 40-plus years Patricia worked with her father, she was right there beside him, assisting him on the Bragg Health Crusades world-wide. They were a team, when you looked at them, you would see only two people headed in the same direction.

Our lives have completely turned around! Our family is feeling so very healthy, we must tell you about it.– Gene & Joan Zollner, parents of 11, Washington

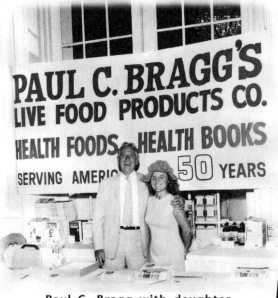

PAUL C. BRAGG'S
LIVE FOOD PRODUCTS CO.
HEALTH FOODS · HEALTH BOOKS
SERVING AMERIC 50 YEARS

Paul C. Bragg with daughter, celebrating here over 50 years of Bragg Health Products, Books & Crusading world-wide, spreading Health around the world.

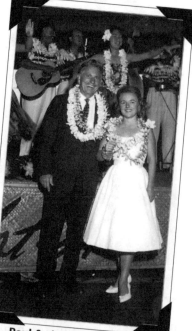

Paul & daughter Patricia, Royal Hawaiian, Honolulu

h

PHOTO GALLERY

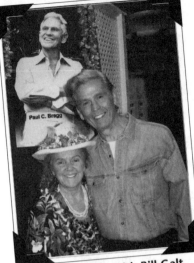

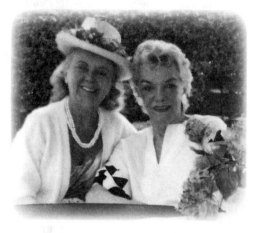

Patricia Bragg with Bill Galt
inspired by Bragg Books and
founded Good Earth Restaurants

Patricia Bragg with Actress Jane Russell.
Photo of Paul Bragg in background.

PATRICIA BRAGG CONTINUING THE HEALTH CRUSADE!

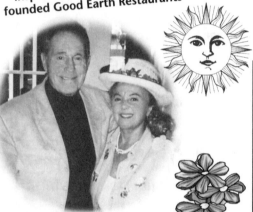

Jack LaLanne with Patricia Bragg

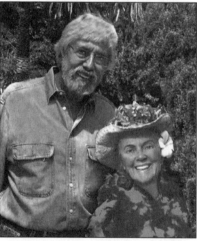

Patricia with Jean-Michel Cousteau
Ocean Explorer & Environmentalist

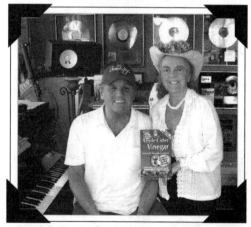

Patricia in studio with famous Beach Boy
Bruce Johnson, Bragg follower over 30 years.
He played for her his latest records.

Dear Friends – you cannot know how greatly you have already impacted my life and some of my friends! We love your Bragg Health Books, teachings and products and are now living healthier, happier lives. Thanks!
– Winnie Brown, Arizona

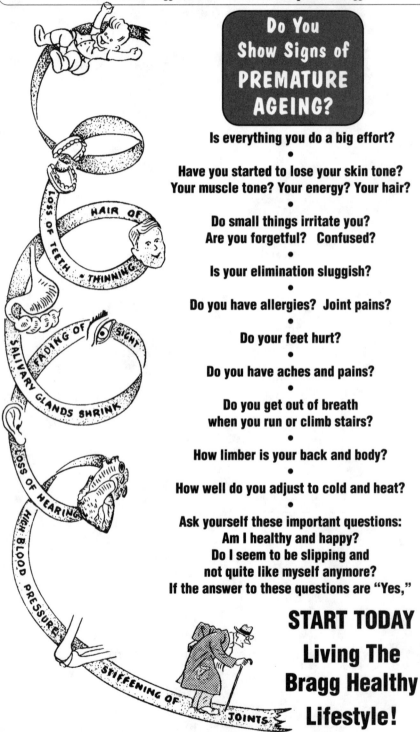

Visit bragg.com and send free Bragg Health Musical E–Cards from our web to friends!
Also follow Patricia and get Bragg Health Messages on twitter.com/patriciabragg
You can watch Bragg Videos on YouTube.com/patriciabragg

Do You Show Signs of PREMATURE AGEING?

Is everything you do a big effort?

•

Have you started to lose your skin tone?
Your muscle tone? Your energy? Your hair?

•

Do small things irritate you?
Are you forgetful?   Confused?

•

Is your elimination sluggish?

•

Do you have allergies? Joint pains?

•

Do your feet hurt?

•

Do you have aches and pains?

•

Do you get out of breath
when you run or climb stairs?

•

How limber is your back and body?

•

How well do you adjust to cold and heat?

•

Ask yourself these important questions:
Am I healthy and happy?
Do I seem to be slipping and
not quite like myself anymore?
If the answer to these questions are "Yes,"

START TODAY Living The Bragg Healthy Lifestyle!

He who understands and follows Mother Nature walks with God.

BRAGG

Healthy

HEART

Keep Your Cardiovascular System Healthy & Fit At Any Age

PAUL C. BRAGG, N.D., Ph.D.
LIFE EXTENSION SPECIALIST

and

PATRICIA BRAGG, N.D., Ph.D.
HEALTH CRUSADER & LIFESTYLE EDUCATOR

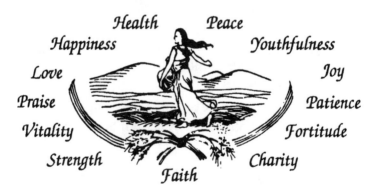

Health   *Peace*
Happiness   *Youthfulness*
Love   *Joy*
Praise   *Patience*
Vitality   *Fortitude*
Strength   *Charity*
Faith

JOIN
Bragg Health Crusades for a 100% Healthy World for All!

HEALTH SCIENCE

Box 7, Santa Barbara, California 93102 USA

World Wide Web: www.bragg.com

Notice: Our writings are to help guide you to live a healthy lifestyle and prevent health problems. If you suspect you have a medical problem, please seek alternative health professionals to help you make the healthiest, informed choices. Diabetics should fast only under a health professional's supervision! If hypoglycemic, add Spirulina or barley green powder to liquids when fasting.

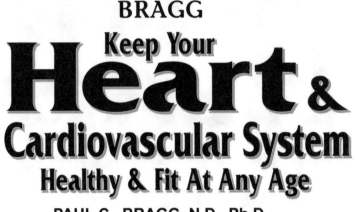

BRAGG
Keep Your
Heart &
Cardiovascular System
Healthy & Fit At Any Age

PAUL C. BRAGG, N.D., Ph.D.
LIFE EXTENSION SPECIALIST

and

PATRICIA BRAGG, N.D., Ph.D.
HEALTH CRUSADER & LIFESTYLE EDUCATOR

Health Science, Box 7, Santa Barbara, California 93102
Telephone (805) 968-1020, FAX (805) 968-1001
e-mail address: books@bragg.com

Quantity Purchases: Companies, Professional Groups, Churches, Clubs, Fund-raisers, etc. Please contact our Special Sales Department.

To see Bragg Books and Products on-line, visit our Website at: www.bragg.com

 This book is printed on recycled, acid-free paper, which saves thousands of trees.

– REVISED AND EXPANDED –

Seventeenth Edition MMXI
ISBN: 978-0-87790-097-9

Library of Congress Cataloging-in-Publication Data on file with publisher

Published in the United States
HEALTH SCIENCE, Box 7, Santa Barbara, California 93102 USA

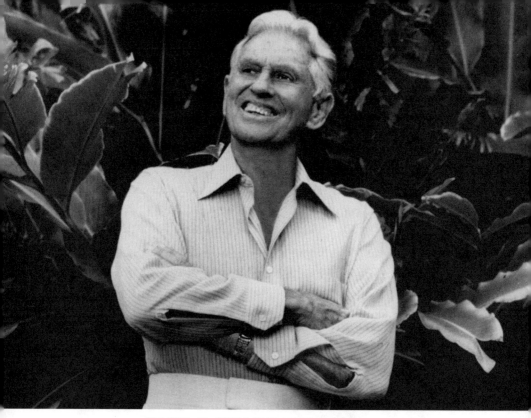

PAUL C. BRAGG, N.D., Ph.D.
World's Leading Healthy Lifestyle Pioneer

Paul C. Bragg's daughter Patricia and their wonderful, healthy members of the Bragg *Longer Life, Health and Happiness Club* exercise daily on the beautiful Fort DeRussy lawn, at world famous Waikiki Beach in Honolulu, Hawaii. Membership is free and open to everyone to attend any morning – Monday through Saturday from 9 to 10:30 am – for Bragg Health and Fitness and Super Power Breathing Exercises. On Saturday sometimes there are health lectures on how to live a long, healthy life! The group averages 50 to 100 per day, depending on the season. From December to March it can go up to 150. Its dedicated leaders have been carrying on the class for over 40 years. Thousands have visited the club from around the world and carried the Bragg Health and Fitness Crusade to friends and relatives back home. When you visit Honolulu, Hawaii, Patricia invites you and your friends to join her and the club for wholesome, healthy fellowship. She also recommends you visit the outer Hawaiian Islands (Kauai, Hawaii, Maui, Molokai) for a fulfilling, healthy vacation.

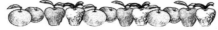

To maintain good health, normal weight and increase the good life of radiant health, joy and happiness, the body must be exercised properly (stretching, walking, jogging, running, biking, swimming, deep breathing, good posture, etc.) and nourished wisely with healthy foods. – Paul C. Bragg

iii

❦❦ *Decades of Amazement as Life Rolls By* ❦❦

Where did our years go? They went by so fast.
When we're young they seem to cra-a-wl,
With each decade, they fly past!

At 29 we're the center; At 30 we feel supreme
But 40 strikes terror; Life's not what it seems.
By 50 we've reached maturity; At 60 we accept seniority.
When we're filled with excitement of creative living,
There's no room for depression and despair!

But at 65, wisdom that comes from experience
Then takes over and we learn to accept ourselves as we are.
Each new day is a gift to be treasured,
Enabling us to go far!

At 75, life is for the living
But it is through our sharing, loving and giving
that we reach the Stars of Joy, Peace
and the Possibilities of Eternity!

– by Ruth Lubin, 88 years young & going strong,
who started writing poetry & sculpturing at 80!
PS: Ruth is a fan of the Bragg Healthy Lifestyle for over 58 years!

❤ WITH LOVE PROMISE YOURSELF ❤

- *Promise yourself to be so strong that nothing can disturb your peace of mind.*

- *To talk health, happiness and prosperity to every person you meet.*

- *To make your friends feel that they are special & appreciated.*

- *To look at the sunny side of everything & make your desires come true.*

- *To think only of the best, to work only for the best and expect only the best.*

- *To be just as enthusiastic about the success of others as you are about your own.*

- *To forget the mistakes of the past and press on to the greater achievements of the future.*

- *To be too large for worry, too noble for anger, too strong for fear & too happy to permit the presence of trouble.*

- *To give so much time to improving yourself that you have no time and no desire to criticize others.*

- *To wear a cheerful expression at all times and give a smile to every living creature you meet.*

– Christian D. Larson
(Science of Mind Magazine)
Author & Inspirational Leader

WE NEED YOUR SUPPORT!

With Your Support The Bragg Health Crusades Can Continue to Spread Paul C. Bragg's Teachings

For over 80 years we have been sharing Paul C. Bragg's teachings on healthy living worldwide! Millions have followed the Bragg Healthy Lifestyle principles and their lives have been changed forever! Everyday people send us letters, e-mails and call, saying – *"Paul Bragg saved my life!"*

Former U.S. Surgeon General, Dr. C. Everett Koop said Paul Bragg did more for the Health of America than anyone person he knew of.

OUR MISSION: To spread health worldwide and inspire youth and people of all ages to achieve optimal health – physically, mentally and spiritually and live long, productive, caring, happy lives.

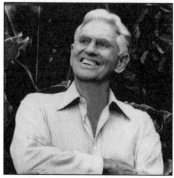

Paul C. Bragg, ND, PhD.
Originator of Health Stores
Life Extension Specialist
Health Crusader to the World

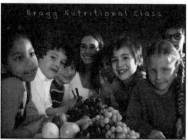

Bragg Outreach to Schools

If your life has been touched and helped by Bragg Health Teachings, please help us carry on the Bragg Legacy into this 21st Century and beyond. Your tax deductible donation to the *Bragg Health Institute* will support our mission to continue the Bragg Message of Health worldwide and inspire future generations.

The non-profit and philanthropic work of the *Bragg Health Institute* funds The *Bragg Health Crusades*, community health, school health education, lectures, seminars, and publications on healthy living. The Institute conducts health outreach to youth in schools, organic gardening teaching programs, and helps sponsor health science research and provides scholarships to worthy students pursuing the natural health science professions.

Please join us in sharing The Bragg Health Legacy!

(Please see next page for more information)

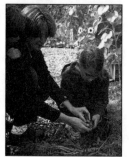

Organic Gardening
Teaching Programs

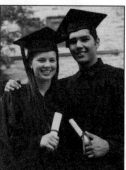

Bragg Scholarships

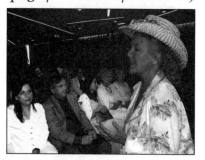

Patricia Bragg lecturing at
Bragg Health Seminars

HEALTH DREAM WITH NEW HEALTH VISION

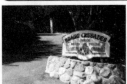
Health Institute Entrance

The Bragg Health Institute is located on a beautiful 120 acre Campus and Organic Farm on the coast of Santa Barbara, California. Patricia Bragg and the Directors of Bragg Health Institute have designated this as the future site of the greatest living tribute to the life of Paul C. Bragg. The new Bragg Health Institute will become a world center for organic and healthy lifestyle education and research. (See our *Mission, Purpose and Vision for the Future* video on *bragghealthinstitute.org*)

You can also be part of Paul Bragg's lasting legacy by having your name permanently inscribed upon one of the educational nature walks or inspirational walls that will enhance the natural beauty of the Bragg Health Institute Campus and Organic Farm. Or you may want to have your name inscribed in the Grand Entrance or one of the rooms in the Bragg Memorial Library or Health Education Center. Your name can be part of your own legacy, as you will be recognized for generations to come as a great Health Crusader because of your financial support of these wonderful health projects. When thousands of visitors see your name each year, they will know that you helped make a difference in the world.

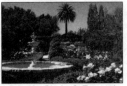
Visitor's Circle & Fountain

Some Special Health Projects You Can Partner with us:

❑ Healthy Lifestyle Teaching Videos
❑ Paul Bragg Library & Rose Gardens
❑ Organic Medicinal Herb Gardens
❑ Scholarships for Future Health Doctors
❑ Special Health Events & Programs

❑ Organic Teaching Gardens
❑ Health Teaching Kitchen
❑ Health Eco Education Center
❑ Bragg Nature & Farm Walks
❑ Bragg Health Museum

— — — — — — — — — — *COPY AND MAIL* — — — — — — — — — — — —

YES! I would like to help support Bragg Health Crusades by making a contribution to the Bragg Health Institute, a 501(c)(3) non-profit foundation, tax ID# 27-0983248 Your contributions are tax deductible.

❑ Enclosed is my tax-deductible gift of $_____ ○ Check ○ VISA ○ MC ○ Discover
  ○ $25 ○ $50 ○ $100 ○ $250 ○ $500 ○ $1,000 ○ $2,500 ○ $_____
❑ Please send me info on where my name can be permanently inscribed at Bragg Center.

My gift is in honor/memory of _____

Please send notice of this gift to (name & address):_____

Credit Card Number:_____ Card Expires: _____ / _____
                                                                month / year
Signature:_____

• _____
Your Name   **PLEASE PRINT**

• _____
Address   **Apt. No.**

• _____ •_____ •_____
City   **State**   **Zip**
• (____) _____ •_____
Phone   **e-mail**

*If giving by check, please make check payable to: **Bragg Health Institute***
Mail To: Box 7, Santa Barbara, CA 93102 USA • (805) 968-1020

vi **For more info check out our web: www.bragghealthinstitute.org**
Spreading health worldwide since 1912

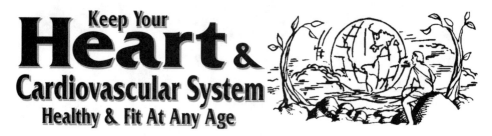

Keep Your Heart & Cardiovascular System
Healthy & Fit At Any Age

To preserve health is a moral and religious duty, for health is the basis for all social virtues. We can no longer be as useful when not well. – Dr. Samuel Johnson, Father of Dictionaries, 1755

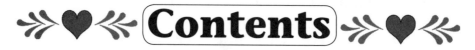

Contents

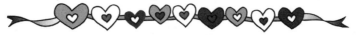

The Bragg Books are written to inspire and guide you to radiant health and longevity. Remember, the book you don't read won't help. Please often re-read our books and live The Bragg Healthy Lifestyle for a long, healthy life!

Kindness should be a frame of mind in which we are alert to every chance: to do, to improve, to give, to share and to cheer. – Patricia Bragg, ND, PhD.

Contents

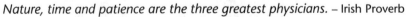

Nature, time and patience are the three greatest physicians. – Irish Proverb

It's never too late to be what you might have been. – George Elliot

Contents

*You can personally significantly decrease the odds of having a heart attack.
It requires changing eating and exercising habits. We guide you in this book.*

A man is as old as his arteries – his river of life. – Virchow

Contents

When health is absent, wisdom cannot reveal itself, art can't manifest, strength can't fight, wealth becomes useless, and intelligence can't be applied. – Herophilus

Cigarette smokers have 50% higher atherosclerosis and hypertension deaths!

Progress is impossible without change, and those who cannot change their minds, cannot change anything! – George Bernard Shaw

*Love doesn't make the world go round.
Love is what makes the ride more worthwhile.* – F. P. Jones

Doubt destroys – Faith builds! – Robert Collier

The better informed you are, the more committed you'll be to making the changes necessary to lower your chances of having a heart attack or stroke.

X

Contents

Energy and persistence helps conquer all things. – Ben Franklin

Contents

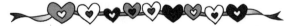

If I were to name the three most precious resources of life, I would say books, friends and nature; and the greatest of these, at least the most constant and always at hand is Mother Nature. – John Burroughs

Contents

Chapter 12: Doctor Healthy Foods 109

The more natural food you eat, the more you'll enjoy radiant health and be able to promote the higher life of love and brotherhood. – Patricia Bragg

Contents

Contents

*Jesus said, "Thy faith hath made thee whole, now go and sin no more."
That includes your dietetic sins! He Himself, through fasting and prayer,
was able to heal the sick and cure all manner of diseases.*

*Enter – or perhaps re-enter – the brave new world of wellness
through exercise, natural remedies, alternative therapies,
prayer, meditation and positive thinking. – Monica Skrypczak*

XV

Contents

Each birthday is the beginning of your own personal fresh new year!
Your first birthday was a beginning, and each new birthday is a chance to begin
again, to start over, to take a new grip on life. – Paul C. Bragg, ND, PhD.

Oat bran is just as effective at lowering cholesterol as drugs
– and many, many times cheaper. – Prevention Magazine

Contents

Chapter 20: Herbs-Garlic-Supplements Nature's Healers . . 199

Your arteries are living structures with vital functions. Their linings have about 98 different enzymatic systems, whose purpose is not only to prevent blockage damage, but to allow oxygen and nutrients to permeate freely through them into the heart muscle and other tissues. – Dr. Savely Yurkovsky, Cardiologist

---

Vitamin E is an antioxidant that helps prevent cardiovascular problems and enhances immune response. It is a primary defender against damaging free radicals. Stores of vitamin E decline with age, so it's important to add ample "E" rich foods to your diet such as: wheat germ, organic whole grains, raw nuts and seeds, beans, legumes, brown rice, cornmeal, oatmeal and sweet potatoes, green leafy vegetables and cold pressed vegetable oils. (See Vitamin E chart page 120)

The use of antioxidant supplements and a diet high in antioxidant foods has been shown to reduce cancer and heart disease and increase life expectancy. – U.S. News/Health Watch

Contents

To maintain good health, normal weight and increase the good life of radiant health, joy and happiness, the body must be exercised properly (stretching, walking, jogging, running, biking, swimming, deep breathing, good posture, etc.) and nourished wisely with natural foods. – Paul C. Bragg

Relaxation techniques are very important health benefits to the body's general health and cardiovascular system. Such techniques as sitting quietly, deep breathing, meditation and ignoring distracting thoughts can bring down blood pressure and are free of side effects. – Harvard Health Letter

Living in harmony with the universe is living totally alive, full of vitality, health, joy, power, love, and abundance on every level. – Shakti Gawain

Life is learning which rules to obey and which rules not to obey and the wisdom to tell the difference between the two!

Talk happiness! Talk faith! Live healthy! Say you are well, and all is well with you, and God shall hear your words and make them true. – Ella Wheeler-Wilcox

Bragg Books are silent, faithful, health teachers – never tiring, ready night or day to help you help yourself to health!

Why My Father & I Wrote This Heart Book:

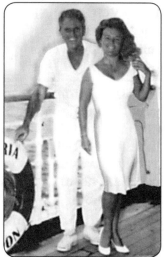

World Health Crusaders Paul C. Bragg and daughter Patricia

Cardiovascular (heart and blood vessel) problems constitute the #1 Killer in the civilized world today. Yet these deadly problems can be prevented and controlled! Millions of our health students around the world have developed strong hearts from weak hearts. Many have averted heart surgery and helped their health and heart by living this Bragg Healthy Lifestyle and Heart Program.

My father, Paul C. Bragg, pioneered these precepts and practiced them for almost a century, with an "ageless" heart in a biologically youthful body even as a great-great-grandfather! We have both thrived on a Diet of Natural Foods all our lives. No salt, no refined white sugar or flour, no artificial additives or poisonous preservatives, no debilitating drinks, only natural "live" foods, fresh organic fruits and vegetables and their juices and distilled water combined with a Program of Healthful Exercise, Fasting, Relaxation and Revitalizing Sleep.

We want to share with you the knowledge we have gained from our years of combined experience and research so that you may no longer fear and dread the #1 Killer. You can choose to be healthy and fit and remain young in heart for your entire life! It's up to you!

❧ ♥ ☙ Bragg Healthy Lifestyle Plan ❧ ♥ ☙

- *Read, plan, plot, and follow through for supreme health and longevity.*
- *Underline, highlight or dog-ear pages as you read important passages.*
- *Organizing your lifestyle helps you identify what's important in your life.*
- *Be faithful to your health goals everyday for a healthy, long, happy life.*
- *Where space allows we have included "words of wisdom" from great minds to motivate and inspire you. Please share your favorite sayings with us.*
- *Write us about your successes following The Bragg Healthy Lifestyle.*

A book is a garden, an orchard, a storehouse, a party, a mentor and teacher. Books can be your guideposts and faithful counsellors. – Henry Ward Beecher

Ask and it shall be given unto you; seek and ye shall find; knock and it shall be opened unto you. – Matthew 7:7

xix

"The best way of determining your individual risk of coronary heart disease is by having a simple blood chemistry profile on a single sample of your blood. This profile should consist of six very important test values: Total Cholesterol, LDL Cholesterol, HDL Cholesterol, Triglycerides, Glucose, CPR and Homocysteine. These tests help save millions of lives by alerting physicians and patients to potential health hazards in time to prevent them from occurring, by making lifestyle changes.

Many leading medical authorities state that all Americans, beginning in their teenage years, should know their blood cholesterol levels, as well as other blood values associated with heart disease! Many pediatricians say from the age of 2 on, children should have their cholesterol monitored once a year by a finger prick test. By identifying heart disease risk factors we can discover problems early and prevent them from developing into costly heart disease in future years to come.

There has been much controversy over the past several years as to what the "normal" vs. "ideal" blood test values should be, especially in regards to cholesterol levels. Listed inside the front cover are what we consider ideal values for the prevention of heart disease."– Dr. John

Dr. John Westerdahl Is A Young Paul C. Bragg Health Crusader

John Westerdahl is a young Paul C. Bragg, for he is a dedicated True Health Crusader. He has spread the message of health throughout Hawaii via his radio talk show "Nutrition and You," and with his lectures and clinics on nutrition, weight control, stop-smoking, stop-drugs and his HEARTBEAT Program which promoted cardiovascular fitness. John's outreach especially in Hawaii has improved the health of thousands.

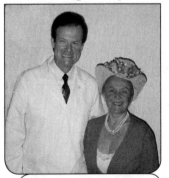

He continues to reach millions with his world-wide Health Crusades, radio and TV shows, and magazine articles. (*bragg.com*)

Dr. John was chosen as one of ten most outstanding young people of Hawaii. He justly deserved this high honor, for he's dedicated and loves being a Health Crusader! We at Bragg Health Science are proud of Dr. John and welcome him as the new Director of the Bragg Health Institute. We encourage more young people into this Wellness Crusade to put America back where we belong, #1 in Health and Fitness instead of way down on the world list.– PB

Patricia Bragg with
Dr. John Westerdahl
Director of
Bragg Health Institute

How to Keep Your Heart And Cardiovascular System Fit at Any Age

Our Active, Busy Life Sharing Health

As health experts and crusaders, we travel throughout the world teaching the simple healthy scientific principles of The Bragg Healthy Lifestyle to millions via the media, TV, radio, and The Bragg Crusades. Every year we would personally interview, and provide Nutritional-Fitness Programs for thousands of people. Among our health students are business and political leaders, stars of the film industry, television and radio, opera, ballet and concert artists to champion athletes, etc.

As health experts, we do extensive research on apples, plants, animals and human nutrition. We also supervise our organic farms and apple orchards in conjunction with the production of Bragg Organic Apple Cider Vinegar. Our writing and working day averages 10 to 12 hours. We enjoy super energy, exercise and tireless, ageless bodies.

Bragg Speaks About His Early Childhood

This robust health which I enjoy was acquired by the methods which are explained in this book. I was born with a weak heart, a "blue baby". Even in modern hospitals of today, newborns with this condition must struggle and fight for their lives. I was born on a plantation deep in the heart of the South, an area where cotton, tobacco and peanuts were grown and hogs were raised.

During the first 14 months of my life there was a constant struggle to survive. From infancy I suffered attacks of heart palpitation. At age 8, it was then I was stricken with rheumatic fever and hovered between life and death for days. My life was not robust, but I had strong faith!

Having heard the word, keep it, and
bring forth fruit with patience. – Luke 8:15

From Degeneration to Rejuvenation

When I was just a young lad I saved a man from drowning. As it turns out this man was very rich and to reward me for saving his life he gave me a scholarship to military school. My parents were very eager for me to attend, so at the tender age of 12, I was enrolled in a large military school in the south (with a high fat, sugar diet). It was at this school that I came down with tuberculosis. I spent time in large sanatoriums, where death sentences were pronounced upon me. There seemed no hope for survival.

But where there is life (and you are still breathing) yes – think hard, there is always hope! I was miraculously inspired by a Swiss exchange nurse at the last sanitarium to go to a famous sanitarium in the Alps of Switzerland. It was there that the renowned Dr. Rollier, who was called the "air, water, sunshine, exercise and good nutrition" doctor, used natural methods of healing to restore my sick body to buoyant, radiant health! Soon I had rebuilt my body and started climbing toward health, strength and energy!

Another important event in my life happened at this time: I made good my pledge to God at 16, that if I got my health back I would devote my life to helping others find the treasure I had found . . . Priceless, Radiant Health! Yes, that was the channel into which I wanted to direct this wonderful new energy and vitality I'd found. So many persons are forever searching blindly for "the light" – seeking health and fitness. Because I had found the miraculous formula of Natural Living, I now desired to pass on this great message to others so that they would emerge from the darkness of sickness into the crystal clear light and brilliance of Super-Health!

For decades my daughter Patricia and I have been researching longevity and natural healing methods. We have brought this message to millions worldwide. The Bragg Crusade has remarkable testimonials of what these natural methods will do to rebuild your total health (see praises earlier pages). We now lay before you The Bragg Healthy Heart Lifestyle based on natural laws and it can do for you what it has done for us and others!

You're a Miracle – Self-Cleansing, Self-Repairing, Self-Healing – Please become aware of "YOU" and be thankful for all your blessings that take place daily!
– Paul C. Bragg, N.D., Ph.D., Life Extension Specialist

xxii

Chapter 1

Your Precious Body
And the Body's Miraculous
Life Pump – Your Heart

Suppose a magician suddenly appeared before you and promised you a marvelous machine which could run itself, direct itself, repair itself, perform remarkable mental and physical feats . . . and would last for about 120 years and maybe more. Would you treasure such a machine? Of course you would! You would keep it in top condition in order to obtain a maximum of service. Every day you would be astonished anew by the performance of this miracle-machine!

True, this is an age of computers, biotechnology and other modern mechanical, scientific and outer space marvels. Remember that the supreme tribute we can pay to any machine is to say, *It is almost human.* Now, stop and think! Our Creator has presented you with the world's most miraculous machine – your own body! This incredible factory has its own *non-stop motor* (the heart), its own *fueling system* (the digestive system), its own human *filtration system* (the kidneys), its own *thinking computer* (brain and nervous system), and its own *temperature controls* (sweat glands), etc. Indeed, this miraculous creation even has *power to reproduce* itself!

Keep Your Precious Body and Heart Functioning at Peak Efficiency

Despite its importance, most of us rarely consider the care of this machine – our body – until illness strikes. By *care* we don't mean *coddling*. Instead, we mean those sensible practices and precautions which keep us in shape for the vigorous daily routine that strenuous modern living requires. Most people are fortunate to be born healthy, but far too often take this priceless gift of health for granted. Unfortunately, Mother Nature does not always let them get away with this carefree attitude. You can ruin a good car by neglect or abuse, and you can do the same with your heart and body!

Unless you know how your body functions – or malfunctions it's difficult to take proper care of it. Most people's ideas about their physical processes are erroneous or far-fetched. Even in this scientific age, too many superstitions and misconceptions about the human body still persist (see page 177-178 – Heart Transplants).

In this book we will explain how the body works, with a straightforward account of the physical, mental and emotional factors which influence it. There will be valuable suggestions on how to keep your heart, body and its entire system running at peak efficiency.

Don't Blame Heart Attacks on Hard Work, Stress, Strain or Tension

You hear a great deal about the modern *rat race* today. You hear people saying that our *mile-a-minute* pace of living causes heart attacks. The words *hard work*, *stress* and *tension* are excuses for the rising death rates from heart attacks. (Reread Healthy Heart Habits – inside front cover.)

The basis for a heart attack is coronary blockage! The question is often asked, *Is there no warning before the blood supply to the heart begins to get dangerously low?* The answer is simple: arterial blockage grows silently and insidiously. There is usually no way of knowing exactly how much and where plaque is accumulating inside one's arteries, usually until it's too late.

In some parts of the body, such as the legs, a reduced blood supply to the muscles can cause localized pain and cramping sensations. The heart sometimes gives angina pain warnings (page 17). Often there's no pain warning. This is why so many fat, flabby people, who eat any rubbish set before them will tell you they are in fine shape (no pain, problems, etc.) without taking special care of their bodies. Unfortunately, many are potentially killing themselves with their unhealthy lifestyle. When the heart attack comes, do they ever blame it on their own unhealthy habits of living? Oh, no! They blame hard work, pressures and tensions, etc!

Unhealthy cooking diminishes happiness and shortens life. – Wisdom of Ages

The Lord gives rest and strength to those who are weary. – Isaiah 40:29

Primitive Humans Lived and Thrived Under Great Pressures

Let's set the record straight: humans have lived under tremendous pressure, stress, strain and tension since the dawn of history. That is what life partly is – a struggle! To live is to exist under pressures of all kinds. Humans have never lived without some challenges even today!

In order to survive, our primitive ancestors lived under pressures that would be difficult for us to handle in today's modern world. Early humans were often the prey of wild animals seeking to kill and eat them. In times of tribal or familial wars, some humans stalked and killed one another. Wind, rain, snow and bad weather would also put them under severe duress. Humans had to survive cruel and vicious natural calamities like floods, tornadoes, earthquakes, hurricanes, plagues, famines and epidemics. In short, stress, strain and tension are nothing new to humanity. Therefore, we believe humans can face and overcome almost all of the hardest pressures life puts upon them if they are healthy, strong of body and alert of mind – this is the survival of the fittest!

The Secret of Survival

Heart trouble need not be an inevitable by-product of mounting work, stress, tension and pressures that people face daily. Though early generations had to exist under tremendous pressure, they were rugged; active physically and mentally. Their secret was simple living, natural foods (without preservatives and pesticides) and ample pure air as well as hard work, which exercises and tones the heart and muscles. As it was in the past, so it is today. Build yourself a vigorous, strong body so that you may face the great pressures of our culture today. Health, strength, endurance, stamina, vitality and energy are your protection from pressure, stress, strain and tension. Face it: this is a tough, rough, cruel and hard-boiled world in which we live. Woe to the weak for they shall perish!

Exercise reduces the risk of heart disease through direct effects on the cardiovascular system and through reduction of intra-abdominal stomach fat. The health goal of exercise and maintaining normal weight is to lower the potential for cardiovascular disease. – American Heart Association (see pages 55 & 228)

Self-Preservation is the First Law of Life

This book is about having a healthy and fit heart and body. All of us must get fit for the long battle of life! There is no substitute for living a healthy life. It's up to you, whether you're rich or poor, to fight for your health and longevity with healthy eating and ample exercise! What do we think of people who sit back and focus on making money for years while they allow their health to deteriorate? Then, when a heart attack or some other crippling ailment comes, they cry, *I have worked so hard! I have been under terrible pressure and tension! All my troubles are due to these strains.* We regard these people as uninformed and their complaints false! If they had given proper attention to their physical bodies they could have had success, money and still enjoyed health!

Hundreds of times we have heard wealthy people say, *I'd give all my wealth for my health!* If they had applied a combination of common sense and a little effort, they easily could have had both! All that is necessary is an elementary knowledge of the workings of the body and its basic needs, combined with the ability to recognize abuse and the willpower to avoid it! People spend years mastering their careers. However, devoting minutes daily learning about the health needs and limitations of their bodies seems difficult for them. **Most people tend to ignore the fact that enjoying well-earned prosperity and long, happy lives depends on their health!**

You Can Restore Your Health and Heart

One of the most remarkable miracles about the human body is its ability to repair and heal itself! For example, if you cut yourself, your body heals the cut. If you break a bone, the body heals the bone after it's set and often it becomes stronger than before. Unexpected injury may happen at any time and to *anyone*! However, if you have been taking care of your body, chances are you will recover more quickly and with less discomfort.

To preserve health is a moral and religious duty, for health is the basis for all social virtues. We can't be as useful when not well.
– Dr. Samuel Johnson, Father of Dictionaries, 1709-1784

The less obvious injuries that we accumulate over time may also be repaired by the amazing human body. After taking a hammering for years, after being totally neglected for too long, *your body can experience astounding recovery and rejuvenation.* You must be prepared to be patient and generous with your time and effort. Just as a business that has been allowed to slip can be rebuilt. So can a neglected body! (See Conrad Hilton Story, page 52.) Don't expect a miracle overnight – *Rome wasn't built in a day.* It takes time and dedication to rebuild broken health.

Coronary Disease is Preventable & Reversible

Dr. Dean Ornish's book *Reversing Heart Disease* states: ***Heart problems are not only preventable, but also reversible by changing your lifestyle.*** (See web: *ornish.com*) We agree – if people would only eat and exercise properly, coronary disease could be stopped in its tracks! Future heart problems would be prevented and heart disease would begin to reverse! People have the power in their own mind to take control of their lives! Most people never know real physical health. They miss out on the priceless benefits of living The Bragg Healthy Lifestyle.

5

Ounce of Prevention Worth Ton of Cure Towards Building an Ageless Heart

Living by The Bragg Healthy Lifestyle principles of proper diet, ample exercise, plenty of rest, and deep breathing, promotes supreme health and longevity. Most people wait until something bad happens to their body before they do anything. We will teach you how to care for your body, so you can have an ageless and powerful heart at any age! Start today – it's priceless, exciting and fun! Challenge yourself – you will rebuild not only your heart, but your entire body!

The Bragg Healthy Lifestyle begins with nutrition. We obtain most of our energy from the food we eat, which has been directly or indirectly acted upon by the rays of the sun. Therefore, a *healthy diet* is important for the creation and maintenance of health. We must not

Your heart takes care of you and keeps you alive, please be good to it!
– Paul C. Bragg, ND, PhD., Originator of Health Food Stores

only eat correctly but also drink the right fluids. Pure distilled water is essential. The next crucial step is keeping oxygen-rich healthy blood circulating throughout the body's great blood pipe system. This is accomplished with daily vigorous exercise and activity. The results will be worth all the effort you put into improving your diet and exercise. Your rewards will be a more powerful heart and a stronger body that can handle your pressures. In the end, you will welcome challenges and your healthy body and clear mind will help you overcome and solve problems wisely and successfully!

Your Health is Your Wealth – It's Up to You!

Health, like freedom and peace, lasts as long as we exert ourselves to maintain it. It's almost exclusively in your hands whether you enjoy a healthy, vigorous life to a ripe old age or live out a half-alive, non-energetic existence with premature breakdown of health. This poor health condition predominates in civilized countries. Therefore, we find it ironic that so-called civilized nations are said to have a high standard of living. In these countries, coronary (heart) disease is the biggest killer! Apparently their high living standards are not producing health and longevity. See revealing chart on page 28. Then start your Bragg Healthy Lifestyle today, to ensure a bright, healthy future!

6

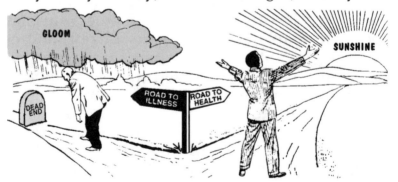

NEGATIVE ⇦ OR ⇨ POSITIVE
The choice of which road to take is up to you.

You alone decide whether to reach a dead end or live a healthy lifestyle for a long, healthy, happy, active life. – Paul C. Bragg

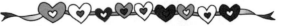

Old age is a highly toxic condition caused by nutritional deficiencies and an unhealthy lifestyle.

One Heart – One Life
To Protect and Treasure

Most people are blessed with a powerful heart at birth. Of course there are always exceptions, like my father, who was born with a weak heart. He needed to fight hard just to survive. But he did survive, persevering to develop a *powerful, ageless heart* for a long, active, healthy life!

Your marvelous heart, the perpetual pump that Mother Nature gives us, can go on beating almost indefinitely. According to Biblical legend, Moses was 120 years old when he died; Noah was 950; Jared lived to be 962; and "all the days of Methuselah" were 969 years. Today, right here in the United States there are over 76,000 people and the count is growing who are 100 years or older. In our research on longevity we have met many people who were 100 to 115 and still living healthy lives. This shows it's possible to enjoy living a long life! What greater treasure and enjoyment is there than a long, happy, healthy, active useful life, and being kind and loving?   7

Truly it doesn't really matter what your calendar age happens to be. In fact, it might be better all around to forget chronological age and consider only anatomical or physiological age. *We do!* Longevity is really a vascular question. *A man is only as old as his arteries.* Sir William Osler, the Canadian medical teacher and writer, pointed out long ago, *"A man of twenty-eight may have the arteries of a sixty year old, and a man of forty may have vessels as degenerated as they could be at eighty."* Remember your arteries are your river of life! Sir Osler stressed the word *degenerated!* Webster's defines degeneration as: *Deterioration of a tissue or an organ in which its vitality is diminished; a process by which normal tissue becomes converted into or replaced by tissue of inferior quality, whether by chemical change of the tissue (true degeneration) or the deposit of abnormal matter in the tissue (infiltration).*

Every day the average heart beats 100,000 times and pumps about 1,800 gallons of blood for nourishing your body. In 70 years this adds up to more than 2.5 billion (faithful) heartbeats. Please be good to your heart and start this Bragg Healthy Heart Program for living a longer, happier, healthier life!
– Patricia Bragg, ND, PhD., Health Crusader & Healthy Lifestyle Educator

Our Miracle Heart and Circulatory System

At birth we are given a heart with clean arteries. It is our unhealthy foods and living habits that cause degeneration. The care we take of our heart determines the number of years we are going to stay on top of this earth. It is up to each and every one of us to take special care of our heart so we can make this life a long, healthy and happy one. Health and happiness go hand in hand.

To understand the causes of heart trouble, we must know something about the heart and the circulatory system. The primary function of this cardiovascular system (heart and blood vessels) is to distribute blood through the entire body, carrying a steady flow of nourishment and oxygen to billions of body cells. Just as important, it is responsible to remove toxic wastes from those body cells.

The blood makes its continual rounds faithfully throughout the adult body's 100,000 miles of blood vessels. These vessels connect to all body cells, from the heart itself, to the scalp, down to finger tips and toes. The average person has between *5 and 6 quarts of blood* continually circulating throughout this network. For heart facts see Nova website: *pbs.org/wgbh/nova/eheart/facts.html*

Important Heart Parts

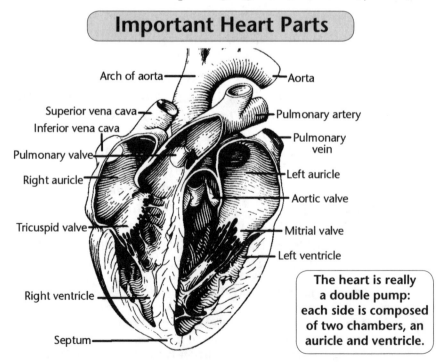

Arch of aorta

Aorta

Superior vena cava

Inferior vena cava

Pulmonary artery

Pulmonary vein

Pulmonary valve

Right auricle

Left auricle

Aortic valve

Tricuspid valve

Mitrial valve

Left ventricle

Right ventricle

Septum

The heart is really a double pump: each side is composed of two chambers, an auricle and ventricle.

Our Heart is a Powerful Muscle

The heart is not an organ of the body, it's a muscle and a very powerful, hard-working miracle! It has to be! *The heart is a muscular (double) pump* whose vital task is to pump the blood and keep it circulating in a life-long journey throughout the body. It's readily apparent that the heart has to be powerful and efficient to do all the endless work required in it's lifetime.

Consider what the heart must do: during rest or inactivity the blood makes one round trip (through the circulatory system) per minute; during activity or heavy exercise it may make as many as 9 trips a minute in order to supply the needed fuel for the increased energy and to remove the burnt-out wastes. Even during rest the heart pumps an average of 1,800 gallons of blood every 24-hours, yet it's no bigger than your fist.

The tissues of the body – including the heart – need oxygen to spark the chemical reaction which provides energy, just as a fire needs oxygen before it will burn and generate heat. The blood's important function is to carry oxygenated blood to nourish all the body's tissues.

The oxygen is first picked up in both lungs, then this oxygen-enriched blood (reddish in color) travels to the heart, from there it is then pumped to the tissues where the oxygen content is exchanged for waste. This blood, depleted of oxygen, turns bluish in color as it makes a return trip to the heart to be pumped back into the lungs.

Thus the heart is receiving 2 types of blood simultaneously:

• supplies of **oxygen-enriched blood** from the lungs and
• **oxygen-depleted blood** from the tissues. To keep these two streams separated, the heart chamber is divided in half by a muscular partition called the *septum*. The left and right chambers formed by the septum are each divided into two compartments. The auricle, which has a thin wall, has little pumping action and serves mainly as a reservoir. The other is the ventricle which has a thick, muscular wall and does the main pumping.

The heart pumps approximately 1 million barrels of blood and beats about 3 billion times during a 70 year lifetime – that's enough blood to fill more than 3 super tankers. – Nova Dateline

Your Hard-Working Blood Network

The object of the blood circulating is to ensure that all the body's cells will be regularly supplied with food and oxygen, and regularly cleared of toxic substances. To achieve this objective, your 100,000 mile intricate network of blood vessels run throughout your body.

Three varieties of blood vessels are: Arteries, Veins and Capillaries. During blood circulation, Arteries carry blood away from heart. Capillaries connect arteries to veins. Finally, Veins carry blood back to the heart. All vary greatly in size, just as do streams and creeks that flow into larger rivers.

The largest blood vessel is the *aorta,* the artery which acts as the main supply pipe leading directly out of the heart and from which – through numerous branches – all parts of the body are eventually supplied with blood. The smallest tubes of both the arteries and the veins are called *capillaries* – they're so tiny that most are only visible under a microscope. Through the body's 10 billion capillaries the last of the food and oxygen is exchanged and the return transfer is made into the veins. The veins then carry the oxygen-depleted blood and toxic wastes back to the heart for purification. On the way to the heart, most of the wastes are deposited in the kidneys for elimination from the body through the urine. Carbon dioxide, another impurity, is expelled through the lungs.

10

For Healthy, Easier-flowing Bowel Movements

It's natural to squat to have bowel movements. It opens up the anal area more directly. When on the toilet, putting feet up 6-8 inches on waste basket or a footstool gives the same squatting effect. Now raise and stretch your hands above your head so that the transverse colon can empty more completely with ease. It's important to drink 8-10 glasses of purified water daily! (More info on elimination on inside front cover.)

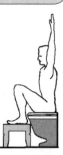

ELIMINATE THE "DRIBBLES" EXERCISE

This helps keep bladder and sphincter muscles tightened and toned for men and women. Urinate – stop – urinate – stop, 6 times, twice daily when voiding, especially after the age of 40. This simple exercise works wonders.

Good elimination is vitally important for your health and longevity!

Blood Purification for Life-Giving Oxygen

When the blood – which is now full of impurities collected from the tissues of the body – returns to the heart through the veins, and then it's pumped out at once through a large artery into the lungs. There the blood sheds the carbon dioxide and absorbs the life-giving oxygen the lungs inhaled. (Don't poison this air with tobacco smoke! Read the Bragg *Super Power Breathing* Book.) The newly oxygenated blood then returns to the heart to be pumped out through the aorta to the body.

Blood circulation is not simple. It follows a design which resembles a figure 8. *There are actually 2 entirely separate circulations, both go away from and back to the heart.* The *greater* circulatory cycle goes to tissues, limbs, internal organs, and back to the heart. The *lesser* one goes only through the lungs and then back to the heart. Pressure in the blood vessels is naturally much greater in the arteries than in the veins, because the arteries channel the blood pumped out of the heart.

A Healthy Heart Has Steady, Rhythmic Beats

The lower part of your heart is slightly to the left side of your upper body, so it's easier to hear the heartbeat by listening on left side of the chest. The heartbeat actually originates in the middle of the neck region and descends from the mid-line into the chest. The heart is in the center of the chest. Myths about sleeping on your left side for fear of compressing the heart is nonsense. The best position for sleeping is on your back. (See page 158.)

A healthy heartbeat keeps a steady pumping rhythm, called the *pulse*. The pulse rate is usually measured at the wrist, where one of the main arteries lies near the surface. *The normal adult pulse rate is from 60-72 beats per minute.* Between each heart beat there is $1/6$ of a second rest, thus when a person has lived for 50 years, their wise heart (pump) has rested 8 of those years!

A low resting pulse rate of about 55 beats per minute or lower rather than 70 beats or higher, indicates that your heart can pump more efficiently.

The heart is made of strong muscles that squeeze in upon itself (contract) with every beat in order to push the blood down to your toes and up to your brain.

Heart rate is high in newborns and declines with age, although heart rate can increase among senior citizens. Females generally have slightly higher heart rates than males. Physical activity can lower resting heart rate, which is important because a slowly beating heart is more energy efficient than one that beats rapidly.

The Heart Has It's Own Intelligent Brain

We often hear the phrase, *I know in my heart it's true.* This indicates that we know that our heart is more than just a pump. It can beat on its own without connection to the brain. It starts to form in the fetus before there is a brain! Scientists don't know what triggers the self-initiated heartbeat. Revolutionary heart research is emerging. I visited the Institute of HeartMath in Boulder Creek, CA. They **found heart has its own brain and nervous system.** In the 1970's, Fels Research Study found that the *brain in the head* was obeying messages from the *brain in the heart.* The heart carries intricate messages that affect our emotions, physical health and quality of life! Our heart has the capacity to *think for itself.* The brain's ability to process information and make decisions is affected by how we emotionally react to a situation. See web: *heartmath.org.*

These dedicated researchers discovered a critical link between the heart and emotions. When the heart responds to emotions such as anger, frustration or anxiety, heart rhythms become incoherent and more jagged; blood vessels constrict, blood pressure rises and the immune system is weakened. Researchers found that many heart failures were precipitated by gross emotional upsets. However, when we feel positive emotions such as love and caring, the heart rhythms become coherent and smoother; thus, enhancing healthy communication between the heart and the brain. Positive heart rhythms produce beneficial effects to cardiovascular efficiency, enhanced immunity, nervous system and hormonal balance. As we learn to become more heart intelligent and improve the emotional balance and heart/brain coherence in ourselves, we will enhance our levels of mental clarity, physical energy, productivity with more daily peace and happiness and a better quality of life.

A key factor in stress is a lack of time. In fact, 75 to 90% of all visits to physicians result from *stress-related* disorders, according to American Institute of Stress. We must utilize our time more wisely, and restore balance in our lives. Researchers found that by *locking in* to positive feelings associated with the heart, such as love, faith, joy, hope, gratitude and appreciation, we can facilitate a more perfect mental, physical, spiritual and emotional balance!

Chapter 3

What is a Heart Attack?

The healthy heart is a model of efficiency and perfection. When people don't watch their diet and don't exercise regularly, the walls of their arteries become cluttered with deposits of a wax-like fatty substance called cholesterol. This damages the arteries, forms scar tissue and traps more cholesterol and also mineral deposits. This condition is known as *atherosclerosis*. Instead of being as healthy and flexible as they need to be for the pulsing blood flow, the arterial walls become hard and brittle, since the accumulating deposits narrow the channel through which the blood must pass. All of this slows down the circulation of the blood and may even cause the formation of a clot, which blocks the blood's flow.

Normal Artery Compared to Clogged Artery

Healthy Open Artery **Cholesterol Clogged Artery**

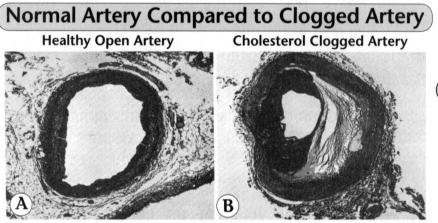

These photomicrographs show (A) a normal artery seen in cross section and (B) a diseased artery in which the channel is partially occluded by atherosclerosis.

When a clot forms in one of the heart arteries it creates a serious condition called *coronary thrombosis*, or *coronary occlusion*. The affected part of the heart is deprived of blood circulation. Failing to get nourishment and oxygen, it then ceases to function. This is when a deadly heart attack occurs. *Coronary heart disease* is when potentially deadly cholesterol-rich plaque builds up in arteries, impeding the blood flow.

Thousands of people every year pay thousands of dollars for state-of-the-art testing to learn their risk for heart disease. However, experts say fresh vegetables and fruits and a health club membership are better buys than any lab test. People who eat a diet low in fat and cholesterol and rich in healthy plant foods, who don't smoke, who exercise regularly, and keep their weight and blood pressure in normal range are less likely to have a heart attack than those who don't, despite any predisposition or genetic tendency toward heart disease. – Harvard Health Letter, health.harvard.edu/

Heart Information by Dr. James Balch*

- **Angina Pectoris:** refers to the pain or feeling of tightness, pressure in the chest. This is a warning sign of impending heart attack. The pain may be mild or severe.

- **Arrhythmias:** electrical disorders that disrupt the heart's natural rhythm. Palpitations happen when the heart beats out of sequence. The victim feels as if their heart is skipping beats. Studies show magnesium can correct irregular heart beats and save lives of heart patients.

- **Cardiac Arrest:** occurs when the heart stops beating. The blood supply is then stopped to the brain and the victim loses consciousness. Unsuspected coronary artery disease is often the cause of these attacks. Victims will experience brief dizziness followed by unconsciousness.

- **Congestive Heart Failure:** happens when a damaged heart becomes fatigued and is unable to pump effectively. This heart exhaustion results in fluid accumulation in the lungs, labored breathing and swelling in lower legs.

- **Fibrillation:** arterial fibrillation and flutter, heart palpitations or enhanced awareness of heart beating. Dizziness and fainting spells often accompany fibrillation.

- **Myocardial Infraction:** blood clots causing a narrowed coronary artery, cutting off nutrients and oxygen to the heart for a period of time.

- **Ischemic Heart Disease:** is caused by arteriosclerosis, in which fatty deposits along the walls of the arteries obstruct the blood flow to the heart. Sections of the heart muscle may die in those suffering from chronic ischemia. It can lead to angina, myocardial infarction (a coronary), cardiac arrhythmias or congestive heart failure.

- **Ischemic Stroke:** A clot lodges in either the carotid artery or smaller artery branching out from it. A clot buster known as Tissue Plaminogen Activator (TPA) is miraculous. It is used by cardiologists, hospitals and emergency clinics! TPA breaks up clots and dissolves them in 71% of patients when administered within 3 hours of an ischemic stroke! Diagnosing stroke symptoms quickly is crucial for recovery!

14

Bragg Health Books were My Conversion to The Healthy Way.
– James Balch, M.D., Co-Author of Prescription for Nutritional Healing

*Excerpts from *Prescription for Nutritional Healing*, James Balch, M.D.

What is a Stroke?

A stroke usually originates from the same causes as a heart attack. The arteries become clogged and narrow because of cholesterol and mineral deposits on the arterial walls, hindering the free passage of the blood. The statement, *A man is as old as his arteries,* is so true and not to be carelessly ignored!

Pressure of the blood trying to force its way through the blockage further irritates the artery walls and creates conditions which give rise to blood clots. When a clot breaks off from the artery lining wall into the bloodstream it can slow or completely block blood flow. If a complete blockage occurs in the vital arteries that feeds the heart muscle, the result is a heart attack or *coronary thrombosis. Cerebral thrombosis* (the most common type of stroke) occurs when a blood clot forms and blocks blood flow in an artery supplying blood to part of the brain (sometimes called *a heart attack in the head.) Cerebral hemorrhage,* a stroke which occurs when an artery in the brain bursts, flooding the surrounding tissue with blood. *Hemorrhagic strokes* include bleeding within the brain and bleeding between inner and outer layers of the tissue covering the brain. *Transient Ischemic Attacks* (or TIAs) greatly diminish blood flow that can last only a couple of minutes and has no long-term effects. *Massive Ischemic Strokes* cause paralysis, difficulty speaking and potentially death. High blood pressure is a major risk factor.

After a stroke occurs the blood supply to a part of the brain is reduced or completely cut off. When the nerve cells in that part of the brain are deprived of an oxygenated blood supply, they cannot function and the part of the body controlled by these nerve cells cannot function either. The brain begins to die. Then your movements can be severely restricted, as well as your ability to speak. The afflicted areas resulting from a stroke depend upon which part of the brain is affected and the seriousness or extent of the damage.

Strokes are a major cause of disability and death among women 50 and older. Strokes can be fatal. It can also produce paralysis of one side or a portion of the body or a single limb. A *lighter* stroke may cause difficulty in moving the arms or legs, in speaking or may result in a loss of memory.

I've seen partially paralyzed people half carried into hyperbaric oxygen chamber often walk out after first treatment! – Dr. David Steenblock, www.strokedoctor.com

Strokes can be prevented by lifestyle changes, health education and faithfully living it is the best protection against having a stroke or any heart problems.

Every year thousands of people become the victims of strokes. Although this disorder is frequently associated with the later years of life, this is not necessarily an affliction of old age. Sadly, this has become an all too common affliction for those in their 30's and 40's. See web: *strokedoctor.com*

Recovery After a Stroke Is Important

After a stroke, the damaged nerve cells may recover or their functions may be taken over by other brain cells. Some victims may suffer serious damage that it will take a dedicated effort to make even a partial recovery. It's important that immediate attention to proper diet and exercise begins! We have seen miracles with stroke victims regaining full use of affected muscles. Speech, massage and physical therapy treatments and hyperbaric oxygen therapy are important and should begin as soon as possible to aid rehabilitation and speed recovery! Prolonged inactivity impairs circulation and makes recovery more difficult. The victim can use his own hands (even if one hand) to massage affected areas 4-6 times daily to bring them back to health. Miracles will happen!

How to Recognize Signs of a Stroke

Ask three simple questions: (1) Ask individual to SMILE. (2) Ask person to SPEAK a simple sentence. (3) Ask him or her to RAISE both arms and stick out tongue. If their tongue is "crooked" or goes to one side or the other, that is an indication of a stroke. If they have trouble with ANY of these tasks, call 911 – FAST! and describe these symptoms to dispatcher. If a cardiologist or neurologist can get to a stroke victim within 3 hours he can usually reverse the effects of a stroke!

Prevention is Far Better than the Cure!

. . . and always more successful! That is why we keep stressing living The Bragg Healthy Lifestyle! You must banish the notion that age alone damages your heart and blood vessels. Remember that age is not toxic. It's not a force, but a measure. Live so healthy that you will never suffer a stroke or a heart attack! You know what your enemies are – tobacco, excess weight, stimulants such as coffee, tea, alcohol and cola drinks, fatty – unhealthy foods, sugars, table salt and salty foods and lack of daily exercise! Take heed, start action now!!!

Patients treated with antibiotic "Minocycline", within 6-24 hours after a stroke, have significantly fewer disabilities, according to this study published in BMC Neuroscience. *Minocycline helps reduce stroke damage by inhibiting white blood cells that can destroy the brain tissue & blood vessels.* – news-medical.net

What is Angina Pectoris? A Serious Warning!

It's when one of the heart's arteries is temporarily deprived of blood and oxygen and goes into a spasm, causing a sharp chest pain! Angina chest pain is the most common symptom of heart disease, especially in women. In the Farmingham Heart Study (see web: *framinghamheartstudy.org*) women were two times more likely to develop Angina pain as their first symptom of heart disease than a sudden heart attack.* This is your heart's warning pain, crying for a lifestyle change to a healthy diet, fasting, exercise, etc. Usually these spasms last only a few seconds, but sometimes 3-5 minutes, and rarely more than 15-20 minutes. These are serious warnings! Please heed these warning signs listed below!

Warning Signs of Heart Problems*

- *Pain or discomfort in your chest, abdomen, back, neck, jaw or arms*. Such symptoms may be signs of an inadequate supply of blood and oxygen to your heart muscle due to potentially serious conditions such as atherosclerotic plaque buildup in your coronary arteries.
- *Nausea during or after exercise.* This can result from a variety of causes, but it may signify a cardiac abnormality.
- *Unaccustomed shortness of breath during exercise.* Although this may be related to respiratory problems (asthma etc.), it could also be a signal of heart trouble.
- *Dizziness or fainting.* This could be a sign of a serious problem – and warrants immediate medical consultation.
- *An irregular pulse.* If you notice what appears to be extra heartbeats or skipped beats, notify your doctor.
- *A very rapid heart rate at rest.* If your heart rate is 100 beats per minute or higher, report this to your doctor.

   *For women the warning signs and symptoms can be different. For more information see pages 38-39.

Some heart attacks will hit strong suddenly, while others begin slowly.

A new paramedic resuscitation method called "Cardiocerebral Resuscitation" has resulted in a threefold increase in survival rates of out-of-hospital cardiac arrests. Most favorable circumstances are when bystanders witness heart attack, call 911 immediately and do CCR until they arrive. The heart is fibrillating (quivering) making it more receptive to CCR and shocks from defibrillator (page 19). The EMS workers also administer vital ephinephrine intravenously as soon as possible.

Understanding Rheumatic Heart Disease

Rheumatic Heart Disease is a condition in which the heart valves are damaged by rheumatic fever. Rheumatic fever begins with strep throat caused by Group A *Streptococcus* bacteria. Rheumatic fever is an inflammatory disease. It can affect many of the body's connective tissues – especially those of heart, joints, brain or skin. Anyone can get acute rheumatic fever, but it usually occurs in children 5 to 15 years old. The incidence of rheumatic fever is low in U.S. and most other developed countries. However, it continues to be leading cause of cardiovascular death in developing world.

The Kidney's Role in Heart Attacks

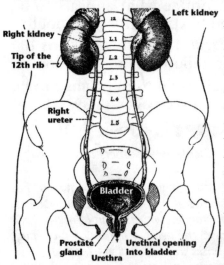

Left kidney

Right kidney

Tip of the 12th rib

Right ureter

Bladder

Prostate gland   Urethra   Urethral opening into bladder

When the circulation of blood into the kidneys is impeded, their functioning is seriously impaired. They are soon unable to efficiently eliminate the built-up toxins that will accumulate in the blood. The body's vital fluid balance then gets upset and sick. This overburdens the arteries and leads to their breakdown. Millions depend on dialysis. Vitamin C and Chelation helps (pgs. 191-198).

18

Be Prepared for Heart Emergencies

Because heart attacks come on suddenly, you should be prepared for such an emergency . . . whether it happens to you or someone near you! *If you have been warned that you are a potential heart attack victim* – it is wise to have a portable oxygen supply, such as *Lif-O-Gen®* with you. It is an investment that may save your life or the life of a loved one! For 15-minutes of oxygen it costs $160, 30-minutes is $300. It is lightweight (3 lbs.) and easily administered.

Everyone should be prepared to aid a heart attack victim in an emergency to call paramedics, fire dept. or life-guards, etc. and give immediate emergency treatment until professionals arrive! Red Cross, fire depts., schools offer CPR and CCR courses, Heimlich Maneuver (choking, drowning, asthma attacks) and other life-saving skills. Such knowledge may help you save lives, also young children have saved lives!

If you witness a person collapse having a heart attack – *American Heart Association* recommends to fast call 911, then start to continuously push hard and fast in middle of chest, ideal 100 pushes a minute with enough force to make chest go down $1^1/_2$ inches. See video: *handsonlycpr.org*. If the heart can be kept going, medications usually help strengthen the heart enough so slowly the body can re-route blood to damaged heart muscle through other tiny vessels. This re-routing miracle process, called *collateral circulation*, helps keep many heart-attack victims alive and recovering!

*IN AN EMERGENCY: *1 teaspoon of* **Cayenne Powder** *in water, or* **Cayenne Tincture** *drops in water helps bring a person out of a heart attack. Also one-half dropperful* **Hawthorn Extract** *every 15 minutes.* Web: healthyhealing.com

Automated External Defibrillator (AED) Offers Fast Miracle . . .

for victims of sudden cardiac arrest. A recent report states that survival rate for those who received their first defibrillation no more than 3 minutes after a collapse has 74%, as opposed to 49%, survival rate of those defibrillated after 3 minutes. The FAA has decided most passenger planes will carry an AED. Med Centers, big businesses, universities, schools, cruise ships, etc. will soon have one in their first aid kits. *www. nejm.org* Medtronic's LIFEPAK® 1000 AED, portable • (800) 551-5544 x41835

Every minute counts! When someone has a heart attack, it's important to recognize what's happening. Immediately get expert help. Calling 911 usually gets paramedics in moments. Do CCR yourself until they arrive. This rapid-response team can provide oxygen, medications (noradrenaline, etc.) on the spot, then patient can be transported quickly to closest coronary-care unit.

Heimlich Life-Saving Maneuver

First Aid for Choking and Drowning Victims and Sufferers of Asthma Attacks

(With the Victim Standing or Sitting)

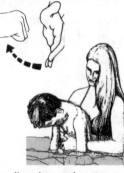

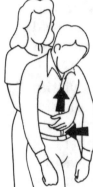

Standing in pool or water, buoyancy of water helps lighten the victim's weight.

I have saved 2 choking victims with Heimlich – PB

20

Save a Drowning victim with the
HEIMLICH MANEUVER
You can't get air into lungs
until you get water out!

1. Stand behind the victim and wrap your arms firmly around their upper waist.

2. Place the thumb side of your fist strongly against the victim's abdomen, slightly above the navel and below the rib cage.

3. Grasp your fist with other hand and press your fist into the abdomen with a quick upward thrust. Repeat until food/water is expelled. Do this more gently for asthma attacks.

4. If the victim is sitting, stand behind their chair and perform Maneuver in the same manner.

5. After victim has been revived and saved, have them see doctor.

Note: If you start to choke when alone and help is not available, then you should self-administer this Maneuver yourself. Many have had too, and it works!

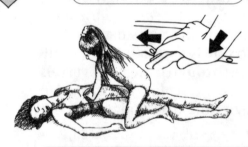

First Aid when Victim has Collapsed and Can't be Lifted, Follow This Procedure:

1. Lay the victim on their back.

2. Face victim and kneel astride the victim's hips and thighs.

3. With one hand on top of another, place heel of bottom hand on abdomen above the navel and just below the ribcage.

4. Press into the victim's abdomen with a quick upward thrust. Repeat as often as necessary.

5. Should victim vomit, (some do), quickly tilt head to side and wipe out vomit from mouth to prevent blocking of throat airway. (Use airway tube if necessary – keep one in first aid kit.)

6. After food, water, etc. is out, it's best a doctor check the victim.

Heimlich Maneuver Jumpstarts Lungs & Heart

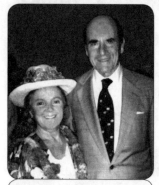

Dr. Henry J. Heimlich with Patricia Bragg in Honolulu

Pioneer Dr. Henry Heimlich, in 1974, developed this technique for choking victims and it has since saved thousands of lives worldwide. Recent evidence shows the Heimlich Maneuver also restores breathing in more emergency situations than just choking. This also helps jump-start the heart in heart attack victims (*heimlichinstitute.org*), and then continue hands only CPR until emergency 911 help arrives. This helps increase survival rate.

Heimlich Maneuver Stops Asthma Attacks

More cases are now being documented of the effectiveness of the Heimlich Maneuver in stopping asthma attacks. As Dr. Heimlich explains, *"We started receiving reports from people who had suffered severe, almost deadly asthma attacks. The people who were with them didn't have any idea what to do. And off the top of their heads, they used the Heimlich Maneuver. They just tried it,"* he says, *"and immediately, instantly a miracle happened, the asthma attack stopped."*

When the diaphragm of an asthma attack victim is pushed up with the Heimlich Maneuver (whether self-applied or not), the lungs become compressed. When this happens, the trapped air is forcibly expelled and the air flow carries away the mucus plugs that started the attack. After the Maneuver, the airway is cleared and the asthma attack ends. Please share this info with asthma sufferers.

When the Maneuver is performed on asthmatics, do it gently, because you are expelling mucus and trapped air – not a stuck food object or lungs full of water. There's good evidence this maneuver can also prevent an asthma attack from occurring. Studies show applying the procedure on a regular basis helps keep lungs free of mucus that can plug up the airway and bring on asthma attack. Please avoid all mucus forming dairy products!

Everyone should know the versatile Heimlich Maneuver, for it is life-saving.
– Dr. Henry Heimlich • Heimlich Institute, Cincinnati, OH • (513) 559-2100
Get radio stations to interview him. (Website: *www.heimlichinstitute.org*)

21

What Can You Do Today to Reduce Your Vulnerability to a Heart Attack or Stroke?

There are many factors which can lead to stroke or heart attack such as: hypertension, smoking, heavy alcohol or caffeine consumption, overuse of aspirin, medications and drugs, heavy fat, salty, fried-food diet and being overweight.

Thousands of heart attacks and strokes occur every day in the U.S.! You could be next – unless you do something about it starting today! You should start immediately to prevent a future heart attack or stroke! The prevention of a heart attack is basically a life-long job of healthy lifestyle living to prevent the slow accumulation of deposits that can clog the arteries. If you are serious about avoiding a heart attack or stroke, you can begin our *Bragg Heart Fitness Program* right now.

Many cardiologists prescribe aspirin for its anti-clotting factor. We don't! They claim it may reduce heart attacks by 30% by reducing blood clotting. Caution: Aspirin may affect natural clotting process too much (a friend almost bled to death). Also, some people develop serious stomach problems and gastro-intestinal bleeding. Instead they need immediate lifestyle changes for a healthier heart! Also, taking aspirin does not lower cholesterol or blood pressure!

The first thing to work for are clean arteries! The inner lining of a healthy person's arteries are smooth and flexible so blood (your river of life) can flow easily.

Importance of Low Blood Cholesterol Levels

Every nation that lives on a modern commercial diet is eating its way into the high cholesterol danger zone of heart attacks. Studies conducted by greatest medical authorities around the world indicates the shocking dangers of high blood cholesterol levels, see recommended levels inside front cover. The U.S. has the highest known average blood cholesterol level in the world, and is generally credited with dubious honor of being the *birthplace of the coronary epidemic!* In fact, 1 out of every 2 men in U. S. will die from a heart attack long before his normal life expectancy. This is a serious reason for Americans to take action right away!

To beat the odds of a heart attack – faithfully live the Bragg Healthy Lifestyle that promotes healthy HDL/Cholesterol ratio and Triglyceride levels.

Americans Love High Cholesterol Foods

Americans love all these cholesterol disasters: steaks, big slices of roast beef, thick slices of ham, ribs, pork chops, fried chicken, bacon, and luncheon meats, as well as cheese, ice cream, whipped cream, cream, sour cream, milk, butter, eggs, commercial pies and pastries, candy, french fries, gravies, potato chips and salad dressings made with saturated oils.

All these favorite American foods have a lot of *hard or saturated fats*, primarily of animal origin. These saturated fats are *high in cholesterol*. Consequently, the average blood cholesterol index in the U.S. today is between 230 and 260 – far above the *safety level*. High blood cholesterol levels have definitely been established as the *forerunners* of most heart attacks.

Remember that the amount of cholesterol in your blood tells you of the risk you are taking of developing a coronary ailment or having a heart attack or stroke. It is *the barometer of your life-span.* It is very important and wise, for every adult to see to it that they do not raise their cholesterol level above a safe, normal level (see inside front cover).

23

Some Blood Cholesterol is Normal

It is perfectly normal to have a certain amount of fat and cholesterol in your bloodstream. Called *lipoproteins,* they are necessary for the upkeep of the body. However, trouble begins when you have an excess of fat clogging your body's pipes. This is why it is essential to master and wisely live The Bragg Healthy Lifestyle; it helps keep your blood cholesterol levels healthy and normal.

Every cell in the body needs some cholesterol to function properly. Cholesterol is not the same as fat. Produced in the liver, cholesterol is delivered through the bloodstream to all the various cells of the body. However, the cells take only what cholesterol they need; any excess remains in the bloodstream. The unused cholesterol eventually collects in the circulatory system as plaque deposits that clog artery walls.

Good news – the liver rarely produces more cholesterol than the body needs. The bad news is that it can enter the body by more ways than the liver's activity. Your lifestyle and what you eat also greatly influences cholesterol levels!

(Recommended Blood Chemistry Values & Cholesterol Levels see inside front cover.)

This fatty substance, cholesterol, is found in the liver, brain, nerves, bile and the blood of all humans and mammals. Eating meat and dairy products (where cholesterol is found) can adversely raise your cholesterol levels. Because when this is beyond the amount your body needs, the excess remains in the bloodstream and collects along arterial passages. *Warning: this arterial cholesterol buildup may cause serious cardiovascular blockage and even death!*

Two Types of Cholesterol – HDL and LDL

Researchers discuss the two main cholesterol types:

FIRST are *high-density lipoproteins (HDL)*, known as *"good cholesterol"*. The lower your total cholesterol level, and the higher your HDL as a proportion of this, the lower your risk of heart attack. The ratio of total cholesterol to HDL should be less than 4 to 1. Researchers believe HDLs travel through the bloodstream collecting *bad cholesterol and disposing of it.*

SECOND are the *low-density lipoproteins (LDL)*, often referred to as *"bad cholesterol"*. When LDLs occur in excess, they can dangerously coat and clog arterial walls, dramatically increasing your risk of a heart attack or stroke. LDL cholesterol is also very dangerous in another way – when exposed to heat and oxygen, these cholesterol molecules slowly change. When this occurs in fats, we call this process *going rancid*. When fats go rancid, their LDLs become infested with *harmful free radicals*.

What Are Harmful Free Radicals?

Today there is much talk about "free radicals" the toxic oxygen molecules that attack the body's cells. These dangerous sources of free radical contamination substances (page 26) cause many health problems and early ageing. The health risk they pose is so great, Dr. Julian Whitaker says:

Free radicals (toxic oxygen molecules), are primary cause of heart disease – #1 health problem facing the world today!
– Dr. Julian Whitaker, Health Newsletter • *drwhitaker.com*

Smoking and obesity lower good HDL cholesterol. HDL can be raised with exercise and foods which are rich in vitamin C. – www.pcrm.org

People who regularly eat barley see significant reductions in LDL (bad) cholesterol, triglycerides & total cholesterol. – Tufts Health & Nutrition Letter

Free Radicals are Cancer Producers

Free radicals are very dangerous elements that can alter and change food molecules. With LDLs (found in all animal proteins and their by-products), free radicals change the original cholesterol structure into more than 400 different harmful, toxic substances! Once in the body, free radicals roam widely, attacking and damaging cells. The free radicals may attack DNA (your genetic inheritance) causing cancer or even birth defects; in the pancreas they can cause diabetes; in the eye they can cause cataracts, and in the blood and blood vessels they can cause cardiovascular disease. Free radicals are introduced into the body through your environment as well as by your diet. Avoid *Free Radical Catalysts* list on page 26.

Free Radicals Cause Premature Ageing

Most risk factors for coronary heart disease, such as high blood pressure or smoking, create free radicals that prevent the inner walls of blood vessels from producing nitric oxide. This is necessary for proper blood vessel expansion and contraction. A free radical is an unstable molecule that reacts with other molecules in destructive ways! An excess of free radicals causes premature ageing and serious medical conditions, depending on which tissues are being attacked.

25

Life-Saving Antioxidants are Life-Savers

Antioxidants are compounds that prevent free radicals from damaging your body! Both antioxidants and free radicals are naturally produced by your body. You can tip the scales in your favor by increasing vital antioxidants in your body through diet rich in vitamin C, E, barley grass, beta-carotene

---

Eating organic green leafy vegetables helps protect against heart attacks. Dark-green leafy vegetables like spinach and chard, yellow vegetables like carrots and squash and yellow fruits like cantaloup and mango are filled with carotinoids, which is one kind of antioxidant. Citrus fruits, including oranges, lemons and grapefruits contain vitamin C, another antioxidant. Nuts, whole grains, oils from soybean, olives, sunflower and corn contain vitamin E, yet another antioxidant. Be sure to eat ample fresh, organic fruits and veggies!

Heavy metals in your body multiply those free radicals chain reactions several thousands, possibly several million times. When a free radical molecule hits a metal atom in your body, the effect is multiplied many-fold. This is partly why it is so important to remove toxic metals from your body.
– www.healingdaily.com/conditions/free-radicals.htm

(found in green leafy vegetables, yams, sweet potatoes, carrots, etc.), and flavonoids (found in grapeseed extract, bee pollen, propolis, milk thistle, ginkgo, etc.). The danger of free radicals is immense, so please maximize your intake of super antioxidants (through healthy nutrition and supplements*) and minimize your exposure to toxic "free radical" catalysts.

Free Radical Catalysts Are Deadly

Don't be a passive victim of destructive free radicals! Take heart, avoid these substances of free radical contamination. Also avoid the unhealthy foods we have listed on page 142. Living The Bragg Healthy Lifestyle helps arrest free radicals and ageing, and earns you a healthier heart and body for enjoying a longer, healthier life! Faithfully guard and protect your precious body and your health! The following substances are dangerous sources of free radical contamination. It's healthier for you to avoid them!

Eliminate Exposure to Toxic Free Radicals:

- **Aluminum** – in antacids, deodorants, baking powder, tap water, deodorants, cans, foils, pots, pans, and in many drugs
- **Cadmium** – most common in batteries, but also found in cigarette smoke, coffee, gasoline, and metal pipes
- **Carbon Monoxide** – auto exhaust, cigarette smoke, smog
- **Chlorine** – tap water, swimming pools and table salt
- **Copper** – tap water, toothpastes and dental work
- **Lead** – dyes, gasoline fumes, paint, plumbing, auto exhaust
- **Mercury** – amalgam (silver) fillings, fish, paint, cosmetics
- **Nitrates and Nitrites** – used in many processed foods, meats, etc. as a preservative. Also found in tap water.
- **Petroleum Products** – fuels, solvents, polishes and paints
- **Pesticides** – Dioxin, heptachlor, dieldrin, and DDT are in most fruits and veggies. This is why you should go organic!
- **Polynuclear Hydrocarbons** – asphalts, fuels, oils and greases. Also deep-fried and char-broiled and BBQ foods
- **Radiation** – environmental radiation, TV & cell phones
- **Synthetic Drugs** – antibiotics, painkillers, barbiturates

---

*SOD, Super Oxide Dismutase, is an antioxidant that helps neutralize free radicals so they are no longer a danger to the body. **Vitamin A** also protects mucous membranes from damage, helps improve night vision, makes bones, gums and tooth enamel stronger and many more health benefits.

Atherosclerosis – A Fat Hardening Disease

The clogging of the arterial system by excess cholesterol – the deposits of heavy, waxy fat on the artery walls – is called *atherosclerosis*. The components of the word, *atherosclerosis*, are of Greek origin. *Athere* means porridge or mush and refers to the soft fatty material in the core of the plaque; *skelros* means hard and refers to the hard scar-like tissue formation involved in the development of a plaque, and *osis* is a greek suffix meaning a diseased condition. Therefore, it's a fat hardening disease.

The term *arteriosclerosis* is a group of diseases that cause thickening, blocking and loss of elasticity of the artery wall. Both atherosclerosis and arteriosclerosis are often used interchangeably. Atherosclerosis mostly affects the aorta – the largest blood vessel in the body, and the coronary arteries and the cerebral arteries which supply the brain, legs and abdomen. Atherosclerosis starts with high blood pressure, smoking and increased concentration of fats in the bloodstream.

Rich American Diet is a Killer

Atherosclerosis is not caused by old age, but by diet! Autopsies of American soldiers killed in battle in the Korean and Vietnam Wars revealed the shocking fact that 77% of these soldiers (average ages 18-22) already had atherosclerosis! In contrast, the Koreans and other Asians who died on the same battlefield, under the same conditions, had only an 11% incidence of this disease. It is well known, the traditional Asian diet consists mainly of rice and vegetables and is low in the saturated fats.

Saturated fats make up 40% of the caloric intake of the average American diet. Most of these are the commercial, hydrogenated fats – the most clogging, deadly of all fats and are not natural in any sense of the word. It's such a solid fat that it cannot be broken down by the body's 98.6°F heat.

The best natural, unsaturated fats break down at body temperature and don't cause clogging problems. These are perishable foods and don't have a long shelf life. In time, unsaturated fats (oils, etc.) can take on oxygen and become rancid, which gives off a strong odor and bitter taste.

Healthy diets leave less room for foods like sugar pastries, cookies, ice cream and candy which can negatively influence your health, weight, blood cholesterol and thereby raise diabetes and heart disease risks!

World Death Rates Due to Heart Diseases from Fat in Diet

Country	Women Death Rate Per 100,000	% Fat in Relation to Total Calories
New Zealand	389	39.8
Sweden	235	39.4
Finland	314	39.2
United Kingdom	354	38.4
Denmark	306	38.3
Canada	229	38.0
Norway	266	38.0
Australia	250	37.9
Germany	299	35.6
Belgium	225	35.0
Switzerland	167	33.6
Austria	311	31.3
United States	323	31.1
France	131	29.5 *
Portugal	312	24.5 *
Italy	213	22.3 *
Japan	161	7.9 *

This chart illustrates the striking difference between New Zealand, U.S. and Japan, the death rate varying by more than 250%. ***The lowest four countries use less saturated fats.*** – American Heart Association

Beware of Saturated, Hydrogenated Fats!

Hydrogenated, saturated fat remains *stable* because it's impervious to oxygen. In reality, it is embalmed fat! The American consumer has been brainwashed by the large manufacturers into believing they are safe and permanently fresh and healthy! A container of this processed fat will keep for years, because it's impossible for it to turn rancid. Clever ads say these saturated, hydrogenated, processed (erroneously called vegetable) shortenings will not smoke. They also make other clever sales claims which have no relation whatsoever to good nutrition. The same applies to unhealthy margarine made to imitate butter. Some vegetable oils are high in saturated fats, as some tropical oils: palm oil and coconut oil. Hydrogenated oils are also high in saturated fat. We use only Bragg's Organic Olive Oil, see video: *www.BraggOrganicOliveOil.com.*

Saturated fats are the hard fats found mostly in animal products such as lard, butter and fatty meat, as well as in vegetable oils such as coconut and palm.

The health and destiny of countries depends on how they eat. – Brillat-Savarin

The USA leads the world in heart disease, strokes, cancer and diabetes!

Animal products also contain substantial amounts of saturated fat, which can cause the liver to produce more cholesterol. Unsaturated fats do not have this effect. Saturated fats are easy to spot – they are solid at room temperature, whereas unsaturated fats are liquid. So, instead of natural, unsaturated fats that will aid health, Americans consume deadly hydrogenated saturated fats, high in cholesterol that coats and clogs the bloodstream, especially the arteries. This clogging eventually can cause fatal or crippling clots (thrombosis) in the bloodstream, causing strokes and heart attacks!

Play it Safe – Know Your Cholesterol Levels

There are many simple home cholesterol tests available. These FDA approved tests are over 97% accurate and require only a fingerprick. The test kit cost between $10 – $20, and is available most drug stores. See web: *testathome.com.*

When you have a complete cholesterol panel ask your doctor for a copy of your HDL, LDL and triglyceride levels (page 45 and inside front cover). These readings determine your main risk factors for heart disease. HDL *good* cholesterol helps protect you from a heart attack. You can help raise your *good* HDL by eating healthy foods, exercising, losing any excess weight and stop smoking. An HDL less than 35 mg-dl puts you at a health risk. The LDL or *bad* cholesterol should not exceed 130 mg-dl. To lower undesirable LDL levels, seek a low-fat, low-cholesterol, low-saturated fat diet. Triglyceride levels over 200 mg-dl, are dangerous and associated with obesity, sweets, fats and alcohol intake.

The American Heart Association recommends the following guidelines to a healthier heart:

- Consume less than 300 mg of cholesterol per day.
- Consume 30% or less calories from fat.
- Consume 10 or less calories from saturated fat.

If you want to keep your daily cholesterol count, purchase a fat gram counter which will help you count your cholesterol, total fat and saturated fat in foods. We personally don't count calories, fat grams, etc. We live our Bragg Healthy Lifestyle and it keeps us healthy! But while you are learning this healthy lifestyle you can count grams if you have extra time.

Saturated fat and trans-fatty acids are the major determinants of cholesterol in your bloodstream, not the cholesterol you eat.

Be aware that cholesterol can accumulate in the skin and tendons, as well as the arteries, to form small flat yellow plaques and lumps called xanthoma. The plaques often found on the eyelids produce a condition called xanthelasma.

Follow these golden rules for maintaining safe cholesterol levels: eat only healthy, natural foods; get plenty of exercise; breathe deeply and fully; drink 8 glasses of pure distilled water daily; get 8 good hours of sleep nightly; fast regularly; and have a positive healthy, happy, mental attitude. Those of you who are at risk of cardiovascular problems – please be aware of your current blood cholesterol levels (see chart on inside front cover).

CHOLESTEROL COUNT OF COMMON FOODS

FOOD FROM ANIMAL Cholesterol Count (mg)	FOOD FROM PLANT Cholesterol Count (mg)
Beef Liver, 3 oz 410	All beans 0
Eggs, 1 whole 213	All fruits 0
Duck, roasted, 3 oz 197	All grains 0
Chicken Liver, 3 oz 126	All legumes 0
Turkey, roasted, 1 cup 106	All nuts 0
Cheeseburger, 4 oz 104	All seeds 0
Ice Cream, 1 cup 88	All vegetables 0
Pork chop, broil, 3 oz 84	All vegetable oils 0
Beef Steak, 3 oz 77	Sources:
Lamb, roasted, 3 oz 77	1. Healthy Eating Club
Chicken Breast, 3 oz 73	www.healthyeatingclub.org
Milk, whole, 1 cup 33	2. www.cholesterolCholesterol.com
Butter, 1 Tblsp 31	
Cream Cheese, 1 oz 31	

10 Foods That Help Lower Your Cholesterol

If your diet gave you high cholesterol, it can lower it too. Here is a list of foods that can help lower your cholesterol:

- *Oats.* An easy first step to improving your cholesterol.
- *Barley & other whole grains.* Delivers soluble fiber.
- *Beans.* Especially rich in soluble fiber, very versatile food.
- *Eggplant & Okra.* Low-calorie vegetables, good soluble fiber.
- *Nuts.* Eating 2 oz. of raw nuts daily can lower LDL by 5%.
- *Vegetable Oils.* In place of butter or lard helps lower LDL.
- *Apples, grapes, strawberries, citrus.* Pectin rich lowers LDL.
- *Soy.* Consuming 25 grams a day helps lower LDL by 5%.
- *Fatty fish.* 2-3 x weekly, delivers LDL lowering omega-3 fats.
- *Fiber supplements.* Psyllium provides 4 grams soluble fiber.

How Much Cholesterol is in Your Blood?

Too many people today eat a diet overloaded with high cholesterol content of saturated animal fats. When these people increase the burden on their bodies by not exercising enough to burn up even the normal – much less the excess – amount of cholesterol as fuel, their bloodstreams become *choked*. Most people know little or care nothing about their cholesterol levels. They merrily go on using large quantities of butter on their bread, toast, potatoes and vegetables. They drink great quantities of milk, gobble gallons of ice cream and eat meat, fish, poultry, eggs, chips, french fries, doughnuts, bacon, ham and sausage – that fill their bloodstreams with excess fat! Little do they realize their high cholesterol levels are leading them to disaster, and they may be literally eating themselves to death! Millions consume as many as 4 or 5 cups of saturated fats daily. Then they wonder why they end up with a heart attack, stroke or other forms of heart trouble – it's clogged arteries!

It has been clinically established that the amount of cholesterol deposited on the walls of the arteries has a direct relationship to the amount of cholesterol in the bloodstream. Thus you can see how clogged the arteries must be when the blood cholesterol level rises to 270, 320, 380 and even higher! Yet these excessive levels are not uncommon today.

Cholesterol and Your Lifespan

One thing that will unquestionably shorten the lifespan is a body that is overburdened with blood fat, an excess of cholesterol! To reiterate: some cholesterol is important to our body processes. The body even manufactures it as extra fuel in emergencies. *Chole* means bile and *sterol* means fatty. Much of the fat we eat is broken down by the liver into cholesterol and excreted into the bile, later to be re-absorbed into the bloodstream for distribution to our tissues.

Experts state "120-180" cholesterol level best: Top medical scientists agree that blood cholesterol level should not be over 180. Some professional opinions . . .
Dr. W.D. Wright of University Nebraska College of Medicine – "150 to 180"
Dr. A.G. Shaper of Makerer College Medical School, Uganda, – "170" best
Dr. Bernard Amsterdam, New York State Journal of Medicine – "180 maximum"
Dr. Louis H. Nahum, Yale School of Medicine – "150" **Dr. William Dock, Professor of Medicine at State University New York,** – "120-180" is optimal normal range.

Sadly, over 107 million Americans have cholesterol levels over 200!

Fasting – Quickest Way to Lower Cholesterol

In our opinion, fasting is the quickest and easiest method of lowering the cholesterol level. We check our blood cholesterol twice a year. If it tops 180, we fast from 3 to 7 days and it soon drops below 150. Fasting (pages 147-154) is an easy way to give the heart and cardiovascular pipes a good cleansing. That's why faithfully each week we fast for a 24-hour period on 5 to 7 glasses of distilled (purified) water and also three Bragg vinegar drinks (pages 140 & 252). For more details on the Science of Fasting, read our book *The Miracle of Fasting*. See book list on back pages for ordering.

Other Ways to Lower Your Cholesterol

Go Vegan: The best way to keep saturated fat intake low and to avoid cholesterol completely is to base your diet on mainly on plant foods – grains, beans, vegetables and fruits. A vegan diet is free of all animal products – this means no red meat, poultry, fish, eggs, milk, cheese, yogurt, ice cream, butter, etc. – this yields the lowest risk of heart disease.

Fiber: Soluble fiber helps to slow absorption of some food components such as cholesterol. It also acts to reduce amount of cholesterol the liver makes. Oat, barley, beans, and some fruits and vegetables are all good sources of soluble fiber. There is no fiber in any animal product.

Maintain Your Ideal Weight: Carrying excess weight can affect one's risk for heart disease. Losing weight helps to increase HDL levels (the "good cholesterol"). People who have a large waistline are at a higher risk than those who carry excess weight around the hips and buttocks.

Blood Pressure is also a risk factor for heart disease and can lead to strokes and other serious health problems (see chapter 4). Luckily, this is another area where we can take control by watching the foods we eat. A low-fat, high-fiber vegetarian diet can help lower blood pressure.

Smoking: People who smoke have a much higher risk of heart disease than non-smokers do. Moderation is not good enough – it is essential to quit smoking! (see pages 71-76).

Exercise: Regular light exercise such as a daily half-hour walk, can cut death rates dramatically.

Less Stress: Getting adequate rest and learning techniques for stress reduction, meditation, yoga, walking is helpful.

Chapter 4

Blood Pressure & Heart Attacks

The Silent Killer – High Blood Pressure

Each time the heart beats, it exerts a pressure on the veins and arteries called Blood Pressure. What happens when you blow too much air into a balloon? If it doesn't pop, the overextended balloon becomes thin and delicate. Properly inflated, the balloon can be safely bounced and moved around. A balloon with too much air becomes a pop waiting to happen. Don't let this happen to your vessels and heart.

We need blood pressure for blood to circulate. Too much pressure makes heart and blood vessels thin and delicate. Increased pressure on arterial walls makes them more susceptible to fatty deposits, and possible stroke or heart attack.

High Blood Pressure is Often Symptomless

The dangers of untreated hypertension can be deadly! If left untreated, arteries can become hardened, scarred, and less elastic, unable to carry adequate blood to the organs. The heart, brain and kidneys are most vulnerable. High blood pressure is highest risk factor for stroke and heart disease. High blood pressure causes heart to enlarge and become less efficient, known as left *ventricular hypertrophy*. This dangerous condition can lead to heart attacks. Many connect stress with high blood pressure. Some studies have suggested chronic stress can lead to permanent increases in blood pressure and heart rate (air traffic controllers who have high-pressure jobs, have a 2-4 times higher rate of hypertension and heart problems).

33

For a healthy, fit heart, it's wise to keep your blood pressure within the normal 120/70 range. You can manage this with simple dietary and lifestyle changes. Exercise, deep breathing, ample sleep and healthy diet helps keep your blood pressure under healthy control.

Don't eat salt or add salt to food, and avoid prepared foods with high salt, sugar and fat contents. Especially avoid simple sugars like refined sugar and *keep your fat intake to a minimum!* Never use highly saturated fats. Avoid the fast, nutritionally empty foods so common in our *rush and go* culture. *Eat nutritious, longevity foods!*

What Blood Pressure Measurements Mean

There are two types of blood pressure readings. *Systolic* pressure (first figure in reading) refers to pressure exerted by the blood while the heart is pumping; this reading indicates blood pressure at its highest. *Diastolic* pressure (second figure) reads the blood pressure when the heart is at rest in between beats, when the blood pressure is at its lowest. Both readings are important; neither should be high. A normal pressure reads 120 over 70 to 80 (120/70-80), with the systolic pressure measuring 120 mmHg and the diastolic pressure measuring 70 to 80 mmHg.

High Blood Pressure in Adolescence

New Millennium Studies presented at the Scientific Session of The American College of Cardiology in Anaheim, California, found that children who are overweight at ages as young as six or seven, are more likely to have high blood pressure by adolescence! Researchers studied 200 children for ten years, examining blood pressure, obesity and metabolic abnormalities. The results showed the body mass index (overweight) correlated strongly to higher blood pressure in the children, even after they reached young adulthood. The finding strongly suggests primary overweight prevention may need to begin even before the first day of school, promoting good nutrition, as well as exercise and fitness.

High Blood Pressure Linked to Mental Decline

High blood pressure can lead to declines in some mental abilities, according to researchers at the University of Maine. Elevated blood pressure is a strong predictor of changes in brain structure and related cognitive functioning. The researchers examined blood pressure and mental function in 140 men and women age 40 to 70 years old. They found that higher levels of blood pressure was associated with greater declines in intelligence tests, visual-spatial abilities and speed of performance!

The large network of veins and arteries through which blood circulates needs to be open, clear and strong to keep your blood circulating. High blood pressure is a sign they are straining, having to squeeze extra hard to push your blood through. This wears them out and your heart, too. Change to Bragg Lifestyle.

Lowering Blood Pressure Reduces Heart Risk

The International Society of Hypertension unveiled results of largest hypertension study ever completed, called Hypertension Optimal Treatment (HOT) study. They found lowering diastolic blood pressure level of 90 mmHg, can help reduce major cardiovascular risk! The study also found that patients with diabetes, who lowered their diastolic blood pressure level to 80 mmHg, lowered their risk of cardiovascular problems. This study amassed 18,790 patients in 26 countries over a 5-year period. According to Dr. Claude Lenfat, director of National Heart, Lung & Blood Institute, *"If physicians lower blood pressure beyond traditional levels of 90 mmHg, there's reason to believe that cardiovascular morbidity and mortality can be diminished."* The study found that patients with coronary artery disease, had a 43% reduction in strokes with those whose blood pressure level was 80 mmHg and lower. High blood pressure (hypertension) is most common heart disorder and leading cause of death in America. Over 400,000 deaths per year in persons age 65-84, are due to cardiovascular disease and more than $403.1 billion dollars are spent for their terminal medical care and fighting for their life!

17 Deadly Daggers of Arterial Disease

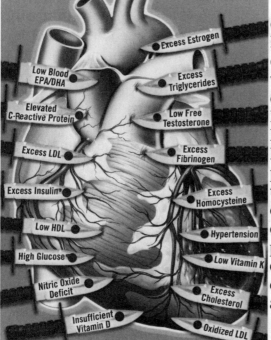

Excess Estrogen
Low Blood EPA/DHA
Excess Triglycerides
Elevated C-Reactive Protein
Low Free Testosterone
Excess LDL
Excess Fibrinogen
Excess Insulin
Excess Homocysteine
Low HDL
Hypertension
High Glucose
Low Vitamin K
Nitric Oxide Deficit
Excess Cholesterol
Insufficient Vitamin D
Oxidized LDL

This heart depicts daggers aimed at a healthy heart. Any one of these daggers would kill if thrust deep into the heart. In the real world, however, many ageing humans suffer small pricks from points of these deadly daggers over a lifetime. The cumulative dagger pricks (risk factors) effects are arterial occlusion, angina or acute heart attack.

Image is from: Sept. 2010, pg. 16
Life Extension Magazine

High Blood Pressure Drugs Pose Health Risks

When it comes to dealing with high blood pressure, most Western doctors turn first to drug treatments. They rely mainly on pharmaceuticals – *diuretics* and *beta-blockers*. Drug *diuretics* (with side effects – see below) lower blood pressure by reducing the volume of blood. With less blood, pressure in arteries decreases. The other commonly prescribed type of drug, *beta blocker,* (also with side effects – see below), works on autonomic nervous system. Beta blockers slow heart rate, which reduces pressure by reducing the amount of blood the heart pumps.

Diuretics & Beta Blockers have Side Effects

These both claim to be helpful remedies for high blood pressure, don't be too sure. **Diuretics** relieve one problem only to cause several others: They deplete blood of certain essential minerals, increase blood's cholesterol level, and increase blood's thickness, stickiness and acidity. These factors increase heart attack risk. Studies show that death rates increase with heavy diuretic use.

What about **beta blockers**? Though their cardiovascular side-effects are less pronounced than diuretics, beta blockers are known for causing impotence, depression and fatigue. Because their job is to make the heart lazy and slow, beta blockers ensure the hands, feet (reason for coldness) and brain get less blood and less oxygen! (*WebMD.com* or *TexasHeart.org*)

You can avoid dangerous drugs and maintain healthy blood pressure at same time. See if changes in your diet and physical activity are enough to improve heart health – just don't rely on prescription drugs. Take advice of a growing legion of progressive medical practitioners who treat high blood pressure without dangerous drugs! Doctors like Alexander Leaf of Harvard Medical School, and William Roberts, editor of *The American Journal of Cardiology*, recommend making lifestyle changes rather than drug prescriptions for high blood pressure patients!

36

Shocking Heart Facts About the #1 Killer

- Center for Disease Control estimates for the year 2010, over 81 million people in U.S. have one or more forms of cardiovascular disease!
- Every 33 seconds an American dies from cardiovascular disease!
- Heart disease doesn't just kill the old; 1 out of every 6 is under 65!
- Heart disease affects both men and women; heart related fatalities are 49% deaths for men, while women account for 51% deaths.
- In 2010 Heart Disease will cost the United States over $317 billion.

Don't let cardiovascular disease affect you! Protect your heart!

What kind of lifestyle changes are best? Those that instill the health habits we teach with The Bragg Healthy Lifestyle! A low-fat, vegetarian diet is crucial for the free and unimpeded flow of blood through your body. Reducing fat in your diet also stimulates weight loss, which, in turn, contributes to reduced blood pressure. Finally, make exercise a fixed part of your daily routine and learn to breathe deeply and relax, freeing yourself of stress while filling yourself with ample fresh oxygen. Begin today to make this Bragg Healthy Lifestyle a lifelong happy habit! It is bringing miracles to millions.

Please listen to Dr. Claude Lenfant, Director, National Heart, Lung & Blood Institute. He says *"Lifestyle changes alone can actually reverse the conditions of heart disease."* (Web: *health.nih.gov/topic/HeartAttack*) When it comes to making the kind of changes needed for healthy and happy living, the truly important thing is making those changes happen. However, actually doing it, living it, making it happen – this is what counts! So don't play procrastinating games with yourself! The moment you think, *Do I have time to do this right now?* is the moment to stop asking and start doing. The moment you think, *I want a big steak for dinner*, is the time to open up Bragg Vegetarian Recipe Book to discover healthy, delicious new recipes. We promise you will find recipes more tasty, healthy and satisfying than meat. If you do eat meat, limit it to 1-3 times a week and be sure it's hormone-free, organically fed without harmful chemicals.

Millions of successful Bragg students will tell you the same thing: the beginning is the most difficult. The in-between moment after you decide you want to become healthier and before you begin to act on that decision, is the hardest. Example: the moment before you put one leg in front of the other on the first step of your brisk walk is the hardest moment of the exercise, get started!

Once you dedicate your life to health you're living The Bragg Healthy Lifestyle – your Fountain of Youthfulness! Soon you will look forward with joy to your daily exercises. Also, you will wonder how you could ever have eaten the unhealthy and unappetizing foods that once half-way sustained you. Plan, plot and follow through with The Bragg Healthy Lifestyle living. Getting started is what counts. Start Now!

Heart Disease in Women: Understand Symptoms & Risks*

Although heart disease is often thought more of a problem for men, more women than men die of heart disease each year! Women are six times as likely to die of heart disease then of breast cancer. Heart disease kills more women over 65 than all other cancers combined. Very few pre-menopausal women have heart attacks, unless they smoke, have diabetes, or are on birth control pills for a long period of time. Smoking seems to be the biggest risk factor (please read pages 71-76).

Women's heart disease symptoms can be very different from the symptoms in men. Fortunately, women can take steps to understand their unique symptoms of heart disease and to begin to reduce their risk of heart disease.

Heart Attack Symptoms Different for Women

It's easy for women to miss heart attack symptoms at the initial stages because the symptoms do show up differently in women than in men. In fact, the top four symptoms are often misdiagnosed. Immediate intervention can mean life or death, so it's a good idea for all women to be aware of the warning signs of heart attacks. Signs and symptoms are more subtle than the obvious crushing chest pain often associated with heart attacks. This may be because women tend to have blockages not only in their main arteries, but also in the smaller arteries that supply blood to the heart.

Many women tend to show up in emergency rooms after much heart damage has already occurred because their symptoms are not those typically associated with a heart attack. If you experience these symptoms or think you're having a heart attack, call for emergency medical help immediately. Don't drive yourself to the emergency room.

*More info on heart disease in women see web: HeartHealthyWomen.org

Women's Health Initiative showed that the chances of suffering a heart attack, stroke or life-threatening blood clot increase significantly within months of starting Hormone Replacement Therapy (HRT).

Research by the National Institutes of Health (NIH) indicates that women often experience new or different physical symptoms as long as a month or more before actually experiencing a heart attack. – see web: usgovinfo.about.com

Women's Symptoms Prior to Heart Attack:

Major symptoms in women *preceding a heart attack*:

- Shortness of Breath
- Sleep Disturbance
- Flu-like Symptoms
- Unexplained Sweating

- Unusual fatigue
- Indigestion
- Pain in neck, jaw, upper back, chest

- Nausea
- Heartburn
- Anxiety
- Dizziness

Knowing these symptoms beforehand, may help women and their doctors identify the early warning symptoms of a heart attack so that they can better prevent the attacks.

Signs & Symptoms During Heart Attack:

Major acute symptoms *during a heart attack* in woman:

- Shortness of breath
- Nausea/Vomiting
- Pain that runs along neck, jaw, upper back or chest

- Cold sweat
- Unusual Fatigue

- Dizziness
- Weakness

Women's Risk Factors are Different

Although traditional risk factors for heart attack – such as high cholesterol, high blood pressure and obesity – affect women and men, there are other factors that play a bigger role in development of heart disease in women. These are:

- **Metabolic Syndrome** – a combination of fat around your belly, high blood pressure, high blood sugar and high triglycerides – has a greater impact on women.

- **Mental stress and depression** affect women's hearts.

- **Smoking** is a greater risk factor in women.

- **Low levels of estrogen after menopause** pose a significant risk factor for developing cardiovascular disease in the smaller blood vessels for women.

Women are at serious risk of heart disease, especially after menopause. In fact, coronary-artery disease is the leading killer of women over 65. Five times more women die of heart disease than of breast cancer. Vital statistics show 53% of women still die of atherosclerotic vascular disease (includes coronary-artery disease, stroke, aneurysms, etc.) compared to 42% of men dying of these causes.

Women should know that not every heart attack symptom is going to be the "left arm hurting". Be aware of intense pain in the jaw. Nausea and intense sweating are also common symptoms. 60% of people who have a heart attack while sleeping do not wake up. Pain in the jaw can wake you from a sound sleep! Be careful, be aware. The more you know, the better your chance to survive. – see web: droz.com

KEEP HEALTHY & YOUTHFUL BIOLOGICALLY WITH EXERCISE & GOOD NUTRITION

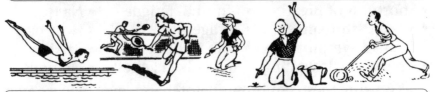

Always remember you have the following important reasons for following The Bragg Healthy Lifestyle:

- The ironclad laws of Mother Nature and God.
- Your common sense, which tells you that you are doing right.
- Your aim to make your health better and your life longer.
- Your resolve to prevent illness so that you may enjoy life.
- Make an art of healthy living; you will be youthful at any age.
- You will retain your faculties and be hale, hearty, active and useful far beyond the ordinary length of years.
- You will also possess superior mental and physical powers!

40

WANTED – For Robbing Health & Life

KILLER Saturated Fats	CHOKER Hydrogenated Fats
CLOGGER Salt	DEADEYED Devitalized Foods
DOPEY Caffeine	HARD WATER Inorganic Minerals
PLUGGER Frying Pan	JERKY Turbulent Emotions
DEATH-DEALER Drugs	CRAZY Alcohol
GREASY Overweight	SMOKEY Tobacco
HOGGY Overeating	LOAFER Laziness

What Wise Men Say

Wisdom does not show itself so much in precept as in life – a firmness of mind and mastery of the appetite. – Seneca

Govern well thy appetite, lest Sin surprise thee, and her black attendant, Death. – Milton

Our prayers should be for a sound mind in a healthy body. – Juvenal

I saw few die of hunger – of eating, a hundred thousand. – Ben Franklin

Your health is your wealth. – Paul C. Bragg, ND, PhD.

Health is a blessing that money cannot buy. – Izaak Walton

The natural healing force within us is the greatest force in getting well. – Hippocrates, Father of Medicine, 400 BC

Of all the knowledge, the one most worth having is knowledge about health! The first requisite of a good life is to be a healthy person. – Herbert Spencer

Chapter 5

Blood – Your Precious River of Life

The body is composed of billions of tiny cells that are nourished by the blood carrying nutrients from the food we eat. As we read in the Bible, *The life of the flesh is in the blood (Leviticus 17:11).* If we can keep the blood in our bodies in perfect chemical balance – so that our vital organs and all the cells of our tissues are properly nourished – and if we keep the pipes of our bodies free from corrosion, there is no reason why we cannot enjoy a long lifetime of *youthful* living. Healthy blood and good circulation are the answers to a long, heart-healthy life free of premature debility and heart disease.

You can start to grasp the power you have to change your health by realizing that *all the red blood cells* in the bloodstream undergo a *complete change every 28 days.* They reproduce themselves about 12 times a year through a series of renewal processes that continue from the cradle to the grave. Our red blood cells are manufactured chiefly from the food we eat and the beverages we drink. If we put the correct nutrients into our bodies and keep our arteries, veins and capillaries clean, open and free from corrosion, we can increase our lifespan to 120 years or more, as expressed in Genesis 6:3 – *May your years be 120!!*

41

Unhealthy Foods and "Dirty" Blood Causes Illness and Premature Ageing

Most humans will not face the realities of life . . . they live in a dream world. When you tell the average sick person that all their physical troubles are due to a "dirty, filthy bloodstream," caused by an unhealthy diet and lifestyle, often they are sensitive and insulted. They want all the modern tests and a specific diagnosis. Then they want a special name and then treatment given to their physical trouble. But they still want to smoke, drink alcoholic beverages, tea, coffee, soft and cola drinks and continue eating lifeless, demineralized, devitaminized, refined, bleached, dead foods filled with harmful, lifeless calories! They want their doctor to instantly banish their aches and pains! How can their physical troubles vanish when the individual keeps breaking important health laws?

The Body's Main Nourishing Arteries & Veins – You Are A Walking, Talking Miracle!

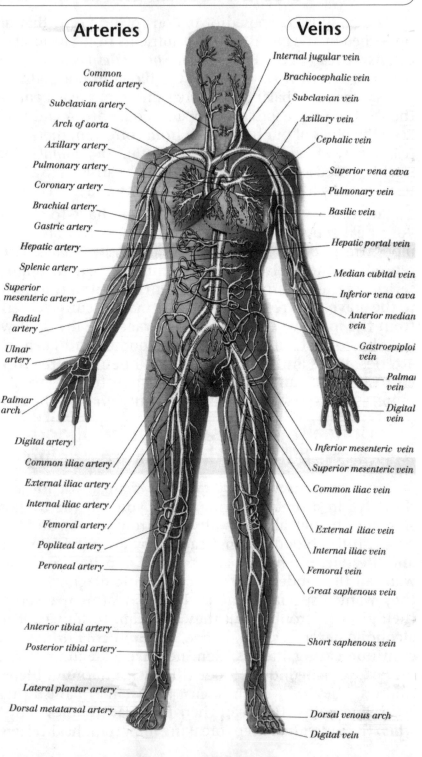

Arteries

Common carotid artery
Subclavian artery
Arch of aorta
Axillary artery
Pulmonary artery
Coronary artery
Brachial artery
Gastric artery
Hepatic artery
Splenic artery
Superior mesenteric artery
Radial artery
Ulnar artery
Palmar arch
Digital artery
Common iliac artery
External iliac artery
Internal iliac artery
Femoral artery
Popliteal artery
Peroneal artery
Anterior tibial artery
Posterior tibial artery
Lateral plantar artery
Dorsal metatarsal artery

Veins

Internal jugular vein
Brachiocephalic vein
Subclavian vein
Axillary vein
Cephalic vein
Superior vena cava
Pulmonary vein
Basilic vein
Hepatic portal vein
Median cubital vein
Inferior vena cava
Anterior median vein
Gastroepiploi vein
Palma vein
Digital vein
Inferior mesenteric vein
Superior mesenteric vein
Common iliac vein
External iliac vein
Internal iliac vein
Femoral vein
Great saphenous vein
Short saphenous vein
Dorsal venous arch
Digital vein

42

Your Bloodstream Carries Your Oxygen

Every one of the over 100 trillion cells in your body demands a continuous flow of life-giving oxygen in order to stay alive, do its job and remain healthy. Red blood cells carry this oxygen via a bloodstream teeming with life. Each of us has between 25 and 35 trillion red cells in our 5 to 6 quarts of blood - millions of cells in every drop!

We have so many of these red couriers of life and health that, in a normal healthy person, the death of 8 million red blood cells every second is not even felt! This is because, in the normal healthy person, 8 million new baby red blood cells are born into existence every second, ready to continue the work of transporting vital oxygen throughout the entire body.

Life Depends On Your Blood Your River of Life

These red cell carriers of the body's oxygen are entrusted with the most important of life-sustaining jobs, but they cannot circulate and distribute their cargo on their own. They are swept along in the bloodstream – the miracle river of life. The red cells and their non-oxygen carrying siblings, white blood cells, swim downstream together in the *plasma* of your bloodstream. Plasma is practically all water; it makes up over half the volume of blood. In addition to the blood cells, plasma carries food, antibodies (for fighting off threatening, foreign intruders), hormones (for regulating body systems) and platelets (for sealing vascular breaks and removing wastes). All the wonders of human life and health depend on blood, it's absolutely essential that you live a healthy lifestyle and keep your precious bloodstream unclogged, and healthy!

43

Blood flow can also be impeded as an indirect result of inflammation. When an artery becomes inflamed, plaque becomes unstable and can rupture, causing the formation of a blood clot – and a subsequent heart attack or stroke.

The heart propels blood through thousands of miles of blood vessels, pumping more than 30 times its weight in blood each minute. Even at rest, the heart pumps over 1,800 gallons of blood a day. For all the work required of the heart, it is relatively small, about the size of a closed fist. In its pumping action, the heart delivers refreshed blood, filled with nutrients (from food you ate) to body's cells through 100,000 miles of adult blood vessels (child 60,000), to maintain your health and well-being.

You're a Self-Cleansing, Self-Repairing, Self-Healing Miracle – Please become aware of "YOU" and be thankful for all your blessings that take place daily!

Elevated C-Reactive Protein Risk Factor

Excess *C-Reactive Protein* in the blood is dangerous. A C-Reactive Protein test checks for inflammation in the arteries. *Chronic inflammation,* is a cause of *atherosclerosis.* Inflammation can be brought on by injury to blood vessel walls, cigarette smoking and high blood pressure. This can cause the plaque present to rupture – triggering clots that might bring on a heart attack or stroke. Studies indicate that elevated C-Reactive Protein may be even a greater risk factor than high cholesterol in the prediction of a heart attack or stroke risk.

There are risks involved when using drugs to lower C-Reactive Protein. We don't agree that people should use drugs when safer, more healthier approaches exist. There are many natural ways to lower C-Reactive Protein.

Safer Ways to Lower C-Reactive Proteins

- **Vitamin C:** Studies show that 1,000mg a day reduces C-Reactive Protein just as well as some drugs.
- **Ginger:** Reduces inflammation, relaxes the muscles surrounding blood vessels and facilitates blood flow.
- **Healthy Diet** is always safer way. Over-eating saturated fat, high-glycemic carbohydrates increases toxic CRP.
- **Fish Oil/Omega-3:** Reduces inflammation in the blood.

Gum Disease Increases C-Reactive Protein

Numerous studies show that people with gum disease almost double their risk of heart attack (see pages 223). These studies indicate that C-Reactive Protein levels decline dramatically when periodontal disease is effectively treated.

Deadly Dangers of Elevated C-Reactive Protein

Studies document *chronic inflammation process* is directly involved in the degenerative diseases of ageing, including cancer, dementia, stroke, visual disorders, arthritis, liver failure and heart attack. Fortunately a low-cost C-Reactive Protein blood test can identify if you suffer with chronic inflammation. We should all be grateful to live in an era when these vascular risk factors can be measured by a simple blood test and corrected before a major cardiovascular event manifests!

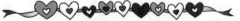

Studies show overweight individuals have elevated C-Reactive Protein Level.

High Homocysteine Levels Cause Heart & Osteoporosis Problems

High blood levels of homocysteine is a marker for heart disease, damaging cells that line blood vessel walls, setting the stage for cardiovascular disease and increasing problems with diabetes, osteoporosis and kidney diseases. When having a physical, be sure blood panel test includes homocysteine levels. Harvard, award winning Dr. McCully says safest and best levels are 6-8 mcm/L. Dr. Paul Dudley White agrees.

For every 10% rise in homocysteine levels, there's an equal risk of developing coronary disease and osteoporosis! In patients with heart disease, the risk of death, 4-5 years after diagnosis, was related to amount of homocysteine in plasma. Everyone produces this substance naturally, a product of protein metabolism. The homocysteine levels rise when body is sluggish and fails to convert it to non-damaging amino acids, then they dangerously accumulate in the blood.

Therapy with B vitamins and a healthy lifestyle menu of fresh fruits and vegetables offers the B vitamins necessary to reduce high homocysteine levels. But a "normal" American diet doesn't supply enough B vitamins to detoxify homocysteine. This has been scientifically documented by Dr. McCully.

45

Thank you, Dr. McCully! Your explanation of the homocysteine theory of heart disease made this a red letter day for me! – Dr. Paul Dudley White's letter to Dr. Kilmer S. McCully, author of The Homocysteine Revolution (amazon.com)

High homocysteine blood levels (safe – 6-8 mcm/L) and dietary deficiencies of vitamins (B6, B12, folic acid & CoQ10 Ubiquinol) are underlying causes of heart, osteoporosis, diabetes & kidney diseases. – Kilmer S. McCully, M.D. (www.homocysteine.com) and (www.drsinatra.com)

Be sure to get enough of the three B vitamins: Folate, B6 and B12.

CAUTION: FDA Approved (harmful) Heart Statin Drug, Crestor® – a drug to reduce heart attack risk by lowering cholesterol & C-Reactive Protein. Unfortunately it has toxic side effects: liver & muscle damage & increased risk of type 2 diabetes. (lef.org)

Recommended Heart Health Tests

- **Total Cholesterol:** Adults: 180 mg/dl is optimal; **Children:** 140 mg/dl or less
- **LDL Cholesterol:** 100 mg/dl or less is optimal
- **HDL Cholesterol:** Men: 50 mg/dl or more; **Women:** 65 mg/dl or more
- **Triglycerides:** 100 mg/dl or less (optimal 70-85)
- **HDL/Cholesterol Ratio:** 3.2 or less • **Triglycerides/HDL Ratio:** below 2
- **Homocysteine:** 6-8 micromoles/L
- **CRP (C-Reactive Protein high sensitivity):**
  lower than 1 mg/L low risk, 1-3 mg/L average risk, over 3 mg/L high risk
- **Diabetic Risk Tests:** • **Glucose:** 80-100 mg/dl • **HemoglobinA1c:** 7% or less
- **Blood Pressure:** 120/70 mmHg is considered optimal for adults

Teenagers Now Susceptible to Heart Disease

Nutritional biochemist, famous Dr. T. Colin Campbell of Cornell University study found that one out of two children born today will develop heart disease, and a new study from the American Heart Association Scientific Sessions *(americanheart.org)*, shows that heart disease actually begins developing early in childhood. Fatty deposits in the coronary arteries begin appearing by the age of 3, in children who partake in a typical American diet - processed foods laden with fats. By the age of 12, nearly 70% of our children have advanced fatty deposits, and by the age of 21, early stages of heart disease is evident in virtually all young adults! Dr. John Knowles, of the Rockefeller Foundation, has cited that 99% of all children are born healthy, yet are made sick as a result of their eating habits! The tender years of childhood should be the healthiest of all, bones are strong, hair is thick, liver and endocrine glands are functioning to full capacity, and they should have inexhaustible energy; yet, their bodies are being fed hamburgers full of steroids, antibiotics, hormones and chemicals; milk that is often indigestible which can cause earaches, colds, mucus allergies, asthma and many health problems.

The latest studies find "adult" diseases are related to what we eat throughout our early years in life. In fact, 95% of coronary disease can be prevented by implementing healthier eating habits earlier in life - reducing dietary fat and consuming more fresh vegetables, fruits and natural complex carbohydrates such as whole grains is very important.

Prevention is important - reward your child for good behavior with fresh fruits, instead of sugary processed candies; establish healthy eating habits before any damage to their health occurs. – Study from: *americanheart.org*

According to the largest federal study of more than 500,000 men and women bolsters prior evidence of the health risks of diets laden with red meat such as hamburger and processed meats such as hot dogs, bacon and cold cuts. The study published in the Archives of Internal Medicine *found that eating the equivalent of a quarter-pound of hamburger daily for ten years, gives men a 27% higher risk of dying of heart disease and 22% risk of dying of cancer; while women had a 50% higher risk of dying of heart disease! Follow the Bragg Healthy Lifestyle to protect your precious heart!*

Childhood Obesity – Huge Growing Problem

A growing concern in recent years has been the increase in obesity among children and adolescents. The problem of childhood obesity is a grave one, in that it can have many lasting effects on one's emotional and physical health! Even back in 2000, it was estimated that about a third of all U.S. children

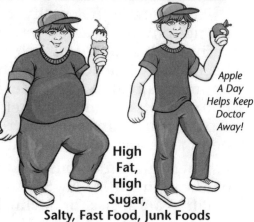

Apple A Day Helps Keep Doctor Away!

High Fat, High Sugar, Salty, Fast Food, Junk Foods

were at risk for developing Type 2 Diabetes in their lifetimes. For obese children afflicted with weight problems, they can develop heart, diabetes, gallbladder and liver diseases, sleep apnea, etc. and even develop high cholesterol.

Studies show children between ages of 6 and 11, the rate of obesity has tripled, according to research study conducted by Centers for Disease Control (www.cdc.gov). More than a third of young people do not regularly engage in vigorous physical activity. Daily participation in school P.E. classes has dropped across the United States.

So why is it that so many children are overweight? The answer is painfully obvious, children overeat the sugar, fat, salty junk foods and exercise too little. Children are driven to school or take buses instead of walking; they then come home and sit and watch ads* for high fat, sugar foods on television. A double whammy! The average American child spends from 2 to 4 hours a day watching TV, playing videos and surfing web – time that could be spent in healthy physical activity. Remove TV and computer from bedrooms, limit TV time.

---

*Children ages 8-12 see an average of 21 TV ads each day for candy, snacks, cereal & fast foods over 7,600 ads yearly, according to recent Kaiser Family Foundation Study. – see web: turnoffyourtv.com/healtheducation/junkfood.html

---

Americans overeat, starting in childhood confirms Mayo Clinic Analysis. They ingest more calories than their body utilizes – jeopardizing health & longevity.

---

*People who eat fast food twice a week and spend 2 and a half hours or more a day watching T.V. have **triple the risk** of obesity when compared to those who eat out once a week or less and watch no more than an hour and a half of T.V..*

Early Lifestyle Can Trigger Obesity & Disease!

Lifestyle triggers obesity in kids. Many young people are not physically active on a regular basis and physical activity declines dramatically during adolescence. Regular physical activity in childhood and adolescence improves strength and endurance, helps build healthy bones, heart and muscles, helps control weight, reduces anxiety and stress and increases self-esteem! It also helps normalize blood pressure and cholesterol levels.

There are numerous reasons for concern for these overweight children. Studies show that overweight children are at risk for having high levels of cholesterol, blood pressure and insulin, making them excellent candidates for conditions like heart disease, diabetes and cancer. A report from Ohio doctors documented 9 cases over 11 years in children as young as 12 years old that had heart attacks that are rare, stated *this is an under-recognized problem*! Pediatricians need to understand that this is a true and real condition! Don't just push aside any child that is complaining of chest pain.*

48

A positive self-image is important for weight control. There are many ways you can help an overweight child regain control of their own weight. By cutting out 100 calories a day, he'll lose 15 pounds in a year! Turn off the TV, video games and encourage more physical activity; sports, handball, basketball, tae kwon do, swimming, trampolining, jump rope, tennis, etc. Teach nutrition and healthy eating practices, not only by making healthy meals, but by your example – eat the right foods and avoid fast foods, high sugar snacks, sodas and desserts altogether. Substitute healthy fresh fruit snacks and raw veggie stick snacks. Eat slowly and chew each mouthful thoroughly. Don't overeat! The Bragg Healthy Lifestyle books inspire and help establish life-long healthy habits for all ages, especially children! Exercising, eating healthy foods, weekly fast day, all helps teach children early prevention to keep healthy and stay fit for life!

*A heart attack in children is typically a crushing-type pain that radiates to the arm, jaw or neck – similar to adults' symptoms. – Chicago, CBS News

You are what you eat, drink, breathe, think, say and do! – Patricia Bragg, ND, PhD.

Control Your Biological "Clock Of Life"

You can only get sound health from your healthy circulating blood nourished by correct food, liquids and air. These substances must be actively distributed throughout your body by the heart and blood vessels.

It is our contention that any person – regardless of age or physical condition – can rebuild themselves and have a stronger heart with cleaner *pipes*. My father demonstrated this with his own body. His abundant health, strength, endurance and stamina were the best proof of the success. He rebuilt his body from a hopeless, physical wreck into a sound, healthy and efficient cardiac machine with vigorous cardiovascular circulation.

Age is not a matter of how many years you have lived! It resolves itself into how clean your arteries are and the health condition of your blood. You can control your own biological *clock of life* . . . and there is no reason why you cannot fulfill the Biblical prophecy:

Man's days shall be 120 years. – Genesis 6:3

"Old Age" is Not Necessary

⟨49⟩

Do not be discouraged by your physical condition! *Remember that the body is self-repairing, self-healing and self-maintaining. Where there's life, there's hope!* Working with Mother Nature, you can start to rebuild a healthy bloodstream, and this will help you build a fit heart. To live long you must have a strong heart and clean blood vessels that are flexible, unclogged and elastic. *This Bragg Healthy Heart Fitness Program is your Blueprint to a New You with vital, fresh Super Health!*

Why grow old? *Old age* is not necessary – at least not as necessary as you may think. Instead of submissively growing old – *revolt! Grow young* – you can defy time! At 60 you can be bright-eyed as a bird and radiate the joy of living. At 70 you can be supple, youthful and full of sunny cheer. At 80 you can wear age like a jewel and who knows, you may become another Zora Agha!

In a Harvard Alumni Study, walking 2 miles a day, 7 days a week, produced the highest protection to stay healthy and not get a heart attack.

You Can "Grow Younger" – It's Up to You

You stand at life's crossroads. Will you take the path of least resistance that often leads to a premature end, or will you climb to the clear heights of a healthful, youthful, radiant life? If you are going to strive for healthy longevity, begin today! Begin right now – don't procrastinate! Regard this Heart Fitness System also as a Program of Inspiration. It's intended to induce you to take stock of your life, get a fresh grip, and hoist yourself onto a higher plane so you can enjoy Health, Happiness and Longevity!

Why not *grow young?* If you have the desire, you will have the power, and by the Great Goddess of Health – Hygenia – you will succeed! Our Healthy Heart Fitness Program shows you how to create a powerful heart, a healthy balanced bloodstream and a strong circulatory system. We can't do it for you – You must!

We offer no *specifics* and no *cures*, for only Mother Nature and God has the power to heal a diseased heart! When you give your bloodstream the proper building materials, you can build a healthier and more fit body to help empower your body to heal you!

50

The Highway to Higher Health and Happiness

Super Health and Happiness! To us, these seem inseparable. Our motto is: ***To make my body a temple pure, wherein I live serene.*** Promoting the welfare of our hearts and bodies is a loving, religious task. By *Health* we don't mean the everyday variety that consists of *not being sick*. We are referring to what we call the *Higher Health* – a sense of amazing well-being that makes a person proud to say with gusto, *I am feeling great today!*

We all agree that the chief aim of life is happiness! There is but one main avenue to happiness that we can recommend with confidence . . . and that is the Highway to Higher Health! Without balanced health – physically, mentally, spiritually and emotionally, it's difficult to have true happiness. The healthy ditch-digger is more in love with life than the sick, flabby millionaire. Great Health is the prime factor in attaining True Happiness. Keep your body healthy and fit and your mind and heart will rejoice!

A Healthy Body and A Happy Mind

A happy and healthy body usually produces a happy, healthy mind. It by no means follows, however, that a happy mind will make a happy body. It would be glorious if the spirit could so triumph over the flesh. But alas the condition of the body usually has greater influence upon the mind, than the mind has upon the body. A person with a healthy sound body and who is spiritual, is seldom miserable, but it's rare for a sick, unhealthy person to be totally happy.

Latest research on a group of businessmen have found that those who had a spiritual connection – attended church or believed in a higher power – had fewer heart problems than those who had no spiritual connection!

3 John 2 is Our Bragg Motto For You
Dear Friend, I wish above all things that thou may prosper and be in health even as the soul prospers.

Studies have also found a strong correlation between personality traits and heart disease. The effects of stress on the heart is more prominent with those who were considered *Type-A* personalities – defined as competitive, aggressive, impatient, and sometimes hostile. Those with *Type-B* personalities are usually more relaxed and unhurried and had fewer heart disease problems. Most studies indicate the shocking facts that Type-A people are twice as likely to have coronary disease than Type-B people.

Lifestyle Changes Help Remove Stress

Stress causes physical changes in the body that can increase the workload on your heart. During times of stress your body releases chemical transmitters that can cause changes in the circulation such as adrenaline and noradrenaline and several types of cortisone. Both adrenaline and noradrenaline have a direct effect on your heart, increasing heart rate and raising blood pressure!

By making positive lifestyle changes, such as deep breathing, prayer, meditation, stress-free walking and exercise, healthy diet, some fasting and a positive attitude . . . this will help you enjoy following The Bragg Healthy Lifestyle for a longer, healthier, happier, stress-free life!

Conrad Hilton Thanks Bragg for His Long Life!

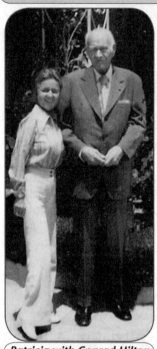

When the world's most famous hotel magnate, Conrad Hilton, was 80 years old and laying on his hospital deathbed, we gave him a new lease on life by introducing him to The Bragg Healthy Lifestyle. He followed our instructions and discovered a whole new healthy, vibrant lifestyle! He was soon healthy, happy and fit, enjoying life! He even remarried at 88 years young! He remained active in business (half days at his Los Angeles office) to almost 100 years young! Mr. Hilton, at 88, was quoted in a *People Magazine* interview as saying, *"I wouldn't be alive today if it wasn't for the Braggs and their Bragg Healthy Lifestyle!"* Here is a photo of the grateful hotel founder with Patricia his healthy lifestyle teacher.

It's Never too Late to Learn and Improve

Men and women today are slowing down the ageing process by living healthier lives. The human structure is mechanically adapted for full energies and activities at 70, 80, 90 and older – clearly proven by the increased numbers of people worldwide who are healthy, clear of eye and keen of mind as they enter their golden years. If you want to get maximum joy out of life, start perfecting your human temple!

This is why we are Health Nutritionalists and Physical Fitness Crusaders. Happiness is largely dependent upon the care we give our bodies. Through harmony of flesh, we achieve the exultation of spirit! Mental serenity is profoundly physical in its source. Through the purification of our body's living tissues we attain a balanced life of Supreme Health! Let's therefore put health of our heart, body and soul first before everything, as everything else depends upon this!

Researchers followed 2,509 people aged 65 and older for 8 years & found that nearly 30% maintained cognitive function. 53% lost some cognitive function & 16% lost lots of cognitive function. People who did better exercised, didn't smoke, seldom drank alcohol, enjoyed work & volunteering. They were less likely to be overweight, not have high blood pressure & diabetes. – see web: lef.org

Chapter 6

The Discovery of Health

Health has sometimes been defined as *physical unconsciousness.* Not all physical unconsciousness is health, but the greatest compliment we can pay to the functioning of our body is to be unaware of it because it is running so smoothly. Most young people do not realize there is such a thing as health because when young, most have it in abundance.

With the passage of years, however, we tend to become aware, thus more *health-conscious.* The adage is so often true that says: *You spend your Health to gain your Wealth.* In later life, its reverse proves true: *You spend your Wealth to regain your Health.* The health-conscious person usually becomes so only after getting sick, and we are of the opinion that most people over 50 are a little sick. There would be no such thing as health if it were not for the lack of it. Most people begin to discover health's existence just when they need it the most. While *health consciousness* may be the result of impaired vitality, let us suggest this applies only to the common variety of health and *health consciousness.*

53

Invest in Your "Health Bank" for Comfort, Health Security and Happiness

Higher Health is essentially conscious or rather, it's the *conscious of its unconsciousness.* It is *health pride – something you should truly cherish.* It's a will and a desire manifestation to live a long, happy, active and healthy life.

Can you think of any greater comfort, security and happiness than that of perpetual sound health? Or that any of your loved ones need never be stricken with an early death from heart disease? Or that no one need die at an early age, unless by an unfortunate accident?

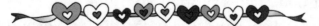

The unexamined life is not worth living. It is a time to re-evaluate your past as a guide for a bright, healthy future. – Socrates

The more you praise, honor, and celebrate your life, then the more there is to be thankful for and celebrate! – Oprah Winfrey

To change the outside, change the inside. – Beatrex Quntanna

Start Investing in Your Health Bank

Perhaps supreme super health seems *too good to be true*. Yet this ideal state of affairs is attainable by anyone willing to apply the principles of our Heart Fitness Program. It is our sincere conviction that the tragic prevalence of heart diseases, as well as many other diseases, is entirely unnecessary and is strictly within one's own control to prevent. Let health become a serious pursuit with you. The time and effort you spend following our Heart Fitness Program will be an investment in your *Health Bank*. This wise investment will bring you and your loved ones great returns in happiness and security. Always remember, *Your Health is Your True Wealth!* This teaching contained in our Heart Fitness Program – if followed faithfully and conscientiously – cannot fail to result in your acquiring and maintaining a more youthful, fit heart. Again, let us emphasize that our Heart Fitness Program does not offer a cure for heart disease, nor can it do anything until it is applied! But remember – the body can do miracles in healing itself if given a chance, as has been proven in thousands of cases.

54

The "Big Three" of Health and Longevity

Suppose you were told that you had to lug an unwieldy load of 20 to 50 pounds around with you wherever you went – walking, sitting, eating, sleeping – all day and all night. How would you feel about it? You would protest indignantly, wouldn't you? Yet that is exactly what you are doing when you are overweight! You are carrying around a load of unhealthy, flabby blubber. You are overtaxing all the functions of your body – especially your heart and circulatory system. Excess fat is dangerous! It exhausts the heart. Insurance statistics show that fat people are the shortest lived. Every pound of excess fat on your body helps shorten your life.

♥ *Rule #1: Achieving and maintaining Normal Weight for a Healthy, Fit Heart*. Normal weight must be attained and maintained by a healthy diet, exercise and some fasting. Forget an operation, they are dangerous!

There is truth in the saying that man becomes what he eats. – Gandhi

💜 *Rule #2: Daily Exercise for a Healthy Heart.*

Vigorous daily exercise helps you to keep your weight normal, it will also stimulate a healthier flowing blood circulation throughout your body. It helps tone your muscles and vital organs, and aids all body functions, giving you the glow of Super Health!

💜 *Rule #3: The most important is Proper Diet.*

A healthy heart and body depends upon a clean, healthy bloodstream, and this depends upon the food you eat! We will discuss all of these points in detail later. When listing Proper Diet as point #3, we are saving the best for last. Your diet is the most important factor in controlling your ideal weight, nourishing your blood and protecting your heart from deadly-clogging cholesterol. Proper diet will strengthen you and make your heart a powerful *fountain of life* and a *fountain of eternal youthfulness.*

Your Body Constantly Works for You – And You Must Work for Your Body!

The body is constantly breaking down old bone and tissue cells and replacing them with new ones. As the body casts off old minerals and broken-down cells, it must obtain fresh food supplies of essential elements for new cells. Scientists are only now beginning to understand that various kinds of dental problems, different types of arthritis and even some forms of artery hardening are due to body imbalances of calcium, phosphorus and magnesium. Many disorders can be caused by imbalances in the ratios of minerals to each other.

Each individual's healthy body requires a proper balance within itself of all the nutritive elements. It is just as bad for any individual to have too much of one item, as it is to have too little of another one. For instance, it takes appropriate levels of phosphorus and magnesium to keep calcium in solution so it can be

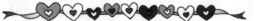

We know that organic whole grains and organic produce contain fiber that's important in lowering blood cholesterol. Diets high in fiber also tend to be relatively low in calories. This healthy eating pattern helps keep weight down and ward off diabetes which is a big heart disease risk in women.

formed into new cells of bone and teeth. Yet there must not be too much magnesium nor too little calcium in the diet or old bone will be taken away and new bone will not be formed. We know that diets that are unbalanced can deplete the body of essential minerals and elements.

Diets high in meats, fish, eggs, grains and nuts and their products may provide unbalanced excesses of phosphorus which could leech calcium and magnesium from the bones, causing them to be lost in the urine.

A diet high in fats will tend to increase the intake of phosphorus from the intestines relative to calcium and other basic minerals. Such diets can also produce a loss of the body's basic minerals in the same way a high phosphorus diet does. Diets that are excessively high in fruits or their juices may cause unbalanced excesses of fruit sugars (pre-diabetes) in the body, which also could leech calcium and magnesium from the body.

Beware of Excess Body Fat

A normal amount of fatty tissue is an indication of health. But when fatty accumulations begin to bulge out here and there and destroy your youthful outlines – beware! These are danger signals warning you that it is time to take action to slim down your excess weight.

Excess weight invites heart attacks: It puts an undue strain on your heart and indicates you have been eating saturated fats that can line arteries with artery-clogging cholesterol. Remember excess fat is fatal to health, youth and makes you more prone to body injury, accident, disease and premature death! (Re-read bottom lines of page 3.)

The old myth that full cheeks and a plump body are indications of health still persists even in our so-called enlightened age. Disease gains a foothold more readily and is more difficult to dislodge when a person is overweight. Fat people have sluggish systems, less energy and endurance! Excess body fat indicates similar excess accumulations around the heart, kidneys and other vital organs, impairing their function and general health.

The Standard American Diet (SAD) is overloaded with too many foodless foods with harmful fats, sugar and salt that raises blood cholesterol levels and raises blood pressure that can cause obesity and fatal heart disease!

Don't Be Overburdened with Fat, It Weighs Heavily on Health & Longevity

To be called fat or obese is an insult which reflects upon intelligence. What could be more unintelligent than allowing your body to be burdened with unhealthy and truly dangerous blubber? It's simply unwise and unhealthy to overstuff your body and burden your heart!

Obese people may be sluggish, tired or slow. Their vital resistance is sometimes low. If speed is necessary, some puff like a steam engine. Their burdened heart and lungs are inefficient and have difficulty handling physical stress. Many obese people move with difficulty. Surplus weight lessens physical activity and often mental activity, too. When an athlete is training for a contest, they eliminate all extra fat from their body. They know that fat lessens endurance and decreases physical energies. This also holds true in the military – maintaining normal weight is a must. An obese man often cannot fight well. Inefficiency and fat go hand-in-hand. They sleep and eat together – but they don't exercise together!

Your Waistline is Your Lifeline, Youthline, Dateline and Healthline

Fat around the abdomen presents more of a heart disease risk than fat on the hips, thighs and buttocks. When you are obese you are flirting with premature old age! You are allowing the old age cells to gather in your body. When obesity happens you are playing with trouble and should be prepared to pay the penalty.

A fit, youthful body must be faithfully maintained. This requires proper care of your priceless human *machine*. The rewards are well worth the effort! If you find fatty tissue accumulating, increase your exercise and reduce the quantity of food you eat and fast one day a week (see pages 147-150 for more on fasting). Don't be satisfied thinking that a naturally fatty surplus comes with advancing years! Beware if you make this mistake, for old age will arrive sooner coupled with serious illness and premature death.

Recent studies revealed fat stored in the body's "spare tire" around the waist increases risk for diabetes, heart disease and serious health problems. Studies say the bigger the waistline, the shorter the lifespan!

Keep Trim, Fit and Your Self-Esteem!

Always fight excess fat as you would your deadliest enemy! It often comes upon you like a thief in the night, silently slowly without warning. Sometimes you realize the danger only when health difficulties are staring you in the face. Then the fight is tougher, but fight you must! Your life may well depend upon your strength and faith!

An unshapely, obese body can destroy your health and self-esteem. You need to be proud of your body, not ashamed of your priceless, human temple. Self-esteem is as necessary to the spirit as healthful food is to the body. If you want to be efficient, eternally youthful, enthusiastic, full of fire and fervor of life, *keep trim and fit and protect your self-esteem!* Build your body as an artist paints a picture or a sculptor molds a statue. Make your body an expression of the best there is within you! Let it reflect your soul and true self. Soon excess fat will find no lodging on your frame and in your flesh!

What is "Normal Weight?"

There are numerous charts, tables and statistics on the subject of normal weight for particular ages, heights, etc. These are based on averages. However, *there is no such thing as an average person.* You may use such statistics as a general guide, but they should not be applied arbitrarily to determine your exact healthiest weight.

If you give your body the proper diet and ample exercise, you will naturally attain and maintain your best personal weight! To weigh a certain number of pounds does not necessarily indicate your proper measurement of waist, hips, etc. If you are firm and healthy – without excess fat – it doesn't matter whether you weigh more or less than the chart *average* for your years and height. The important thing is to find your own best weight as the result of proper care you give your body. If your body is healthy, trim and fit, then your weight is normal for you. *Remember that excess flabby fat is never normal!*

It's a lean, fit horse for the long, healthy successful race of life! – Paul C. Bragg

He who cannot find time for exercise, will have to find time for illness. – Derby

Study Shows Being Fit Saves You Money

Back in 2005 the average American spent $6,683 a year on health care. By year 2015, cost will rise to over $12,320. The Center for Disease Control (CDC) reports that obesity cost U.S. estimated $117 billion back in 2000. It is estimated direct medical costs related to physical inactivity are about $76 billion. A study done by Dr. Ted Mitchell of The Cooper Clinic in Texas monitored 6,679 men. Results showed those who exercised more, required fewer doctor visits. Being fit can cut yearly medical expenses by 25 to 60%. This study also found all you need to stay fit is to exercise just 20 to 30 minutes a day, four or five days a week. Physically fit people live longer and enjoy a better quality of life! Visit website: *cooperaerobics.com*

Be Your Body's Health Captain

You must not be a slave to any bad habits that will damage your heart or body and contribute to a heart attack or illness. That goes not only for tobacco, but coffee, caffeine teas, drugs, alcohol, salt and saturated fats. Look at these poisons as your heart's enemies! For a strong, healthy heart you must faithfully practice Health Mindedness. In your mind's eye see yourself as you wish to be – strong, healthy and youthful. A person in charge of his body is not a slave to unhealthy lifestyle habits!

Free yourself from bondage of these killing habits:
- ❤ "I will not use tobacco."   ❤ "I will not over-eat."
- ❤ "I will not drink black tea."   ❤ "I will not use salt."
- ❤ "I will not drink coffee, sodas and alcoholic drinks."
- ❤ "I will not clog my arteries with saturated fats."

Habits that destroy the health of your body must be broken with strong willpower! Say to yourself repeatedly and believe it, that your intelligent mind will health captain your body towards super health! Let no person or circumstances break your iron willpower! Let no one brainwash you! You must do your own thinking! You can and will control your own mind, body and health. With inner strength you can break all your bad habits!

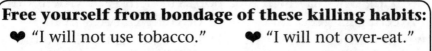

Ten Little, Two-Letter Words of Action To Say Daily:
If it is to be, it is up to me!

Be your own health captain and do what needs to be done for your health!

Coffee and Non-Herbal Teas are Drugs

Coffee is a harmful stimulant to the heart. It contains the drug caffeine which makes the heart beat faster and puts it under an undue, unhealthy strain. Coffee also contains tars and acids which are injurious to the heart, blood vessels and other tissues. These same agents are also present in decaffeinated coffee. Don't drink coffee – it has no nutrients and no vitamins or minerals! Coffee is worthless and harmful to your health! The same goes for non-herbal teas. Don't contaminate blood with toxins – black teas also contain tannic acid that's used to cure shoe leather!

Study Shows Cola Drinks Toxic To Body

What do cola drinks contain? Three toxic stimulants and carbonated water! Colas contain caffeine, phosphoric acid and refined white sugar (also some diet colas contain toxic aspartame, page 62); all are toxic empty calories without any health nutrient value. They also contain carbonated water, which irritates the kidneys and liver! *Recent study says: Don't drink colas or any sodas – and don't let your children ruin their health with these drinks!* According to Center for Science in the Public Interest, the average American teenager is drinking twice as much soda pop as back in 1974. One-fourth of teenagers get 25% or more of their calories from soda, which is filled with sugar. In fact, teens consume 2 to 3 times as much sugar than U.S. government guidelines! New study links increased soda consumption to heart disease, diabetes, obesity, flatulence, kidney stones and calcium deficiency.

60

Caffeine is a Dangerous Habit: How much coffee do you drink?
Research found that 12% of Americans have 1-2 cups daily; 17% – 3-4 cups; 15% – 5-6 cups; 10% – 7-8 cups; 12% – 8 or more cups and 17% no coffee at all.
Don't use coffee and caffeine products if you want super health!

Coffee increases the toxic free fatty acid levels in blood that causes degenerative diseases! "There is a strong likelihood that coffee and caffeine may prove to be one of the most dangerous toxins to human life." – Cancer Research

The digestive organs of coffee drinkers are in a state of chronic derangement which reacts on the brain, producing fretful moods. – Dr. Bock, 1910

Caffeine: *Increases blood pressure, depletes calcium & magnesium from body, elevates cholesterol levels & increases level of dangerous homocysteine in blood. When your coffee high wears off, you feel the drop in terms of fatigue, irritability, headache & confusion. – Caffeine Blues, Stephen Cherniske, M.S. (amazon.com).*

Alcohol is a Depressant and a Killer!

Alcohol, generally considered a stimulant, is actually a depressant. It dilates the blood vessels, in time breaking the tiny capillaries, especially of the nose, cheeks, neck and ankles (example: red, swollen nose of hard drinkers). Alcohol is also a relaxant, dulls and paralyses the brain. The drinker loses good judgement and control of the body and the brain becomes confused. This is therefore the cause of millions of car accidents, crimes, killings, rapes, fights and unnecessary deaths. *Drinking alcohol is so dangerous, an unhealthy way to relax!*

The chief toxic effect of alcohol is on the brain and nervous system! Alcohol *burns up* by depleting the body of vitamin C and also B (the essential nerve vitamin). This, in combination with capillary dilation, can lead to brain hemorrhaging – which in turn, can lead to paralysis. Medical research has shown that the boisterous actions, loud speech, joviality, bravado and *devil-may-care* attitude of the alcoholic are actually the beginning paralysis of certain parts of the brain! Visit: *alcoholics-anonymous.org*

Stay away from dangerous alcohol!! It is nothing but *empty calories*. It will burden your body with unhealthy, flabby fat, in addition to its other toxic, poisonous and injurious effects. The *numbing effect of alcohol* on the pain centers of the brain and nervous system is a *special danger to anyone with a heart condition*. Without being alert to Mother Nature's warning signal – pain – a heart attack, which could be averted when action is taken, may prove fatal!

Say "No" to Self-Drugging Ads!

If you try the TV drugs for yourself, the side-effects and long-term results could be serious! Even though constant TV ads keep telling us what to take to solve aches, pains, upset stomachs, insomnia, etc., plus side-effects. It's wise to seek advice from alternative health care advisors and follow directions exactly and daily monitor results!

The alcohol habit is the most harmful to the body and heart and must be stopped! The Center for Disease Control & Prevention states excessive alcohol consumption is 3rd largest cause of death, after smoking and obesity. Alcohol fosters body cancer and even moderate drinking is risky to your health!

Beware of Toxic, Deadly Aspartame and Chemical Sugar Substitutes!

Although its name sounds "tame," this deadly neurotoxin is anything but! Aspartame is an artificial sweetener (over 200 times sweeter than sugar) made by Monsanto Corporation and marketed as "Nutrasweet," "Equal," "Spoonful," and countless other trade names. Although aspartame is added to over 9,000 food products, it is not fit for human consumption! This toxic poison changes into formaldehyde in the body and has been linked to migraines, seizures, vision loss and symptoms relating to Lupus, Parkinson's Disease, Multiple Sclerosis and other health destroying conditions. Besides being a deadly poison, aspartame actually contributes to weight gain by causing a craving for carbohydrates. A study of 80,000 women by American Cancer Society found those who used this toxic "diet" sweetener actually gained more weight than those who didn't use aspartame products. To learn more about the deadly health risks and crime against our precious health, check web: *aspartamekills.com*

High Fructose Corn Syrup (HFCS) is a highly processed sugar that contains similar amounts of unbound fructose and glucose. What makes HFCS unhealthy is that it is metabolized to fat in your body far more rapidly than any other sugar. It is a primary factor behind a number of health epidemics, including obesity, diabetes and heart disease.

STEVIA – World's Healthiest Sweetener

Stevia, an herbal sweetener, is a healthy alternative for diabetics. Stevia drops (2 drops =1 tsp sugar) from a South African plant, helps regulate blood sugar and lowers blood pressure, but doesn't affect normal blood pressure. Calorie-free Stevia (drops or powder) is suitable for diabetics, safe for children, doesn't cause cavities. It helps mental alertness, combats fatigue and improves digestion. See web: *stevia.com*

High sugar consumption can overstimulate and harm your whole body system, and can lead to many serious health problems, ranging from obesity, cancer, and heart trouble, to high blood sugar levels and diabetes.

More than 21 million American adults and children suffer from Type 2 Diabetes. Simply adding a quarter-teaspoon of cinnamon a day to your diet can safely drop blood sugar levels! Bragg Organic Raw Apple Cider Vinegar with the "mother enzyme" also helps lower glucose levels. See web: bragg.com

Chapter 7

Doctor Human Mind

A Sound Mind in a Sound, Healthy Body

Shakespeare, almost 400 years ago, anticipated the dominant psychology of our time when he said, *It is the mind that makes a body rich.* It's true that the mind guides the body. Likewise, the body helps the mind and links us to the Infinite Spirit of Life! When we are truly healthy, we are brim full in body, mind and spirit (3 John 2).

Our body relates us to the Universe in which we live – the Earth. We are related to Mother Earth through the food we eat, the water we drink, the air we breathe and the sunshine that warms us with its all-pervading power. All are essential for a healthy body and to the continuance of our life! All these nurturing things we need in as pure a form as Mother Nature and God have provided them, without depleting or denaturing them.

The food we eat is related to our daily health. Our bloodstream's system carries essential nutrients that provide the energy and vitality for the functioning of every part of the body. What we eat at this hour today will be nourishment in our cells within 24 hours.

If we eat organic foods as Mother Nature prepared it with her own unmatched chemistry and without losing essential elements – then it will meet our requirements for the growth, health and chemical balance of the body. It will build a powerful, long lasting, strong heart for you. It will give you an alert and active mind. Healthy foods will add life to your years – and years to your life!

Thy food shall be thy remedy. – Hippocrates, Father of Medicine, 400 B.C.

Beloved, I wish above all things that thou may prosper and be in health, even as thy soul prospers. – 3 John 2

Forgive and forget is the best advice for a healthy heart. Holding onto vengeful thoughts, grudges and jealousy can increase your blood pressure, heart rate and muscle tension. Anger can actually thicken your blood and increase your risk for strokes and heart problems! – Natural Health

A fool thinks he needs no advice, but a wise man listens to others. – Proverbs 12:15

Correct Thinking is Important for Health

In the Book of Life, the Bible, Proverbs 23:7 tells us:
For as he thinketh in his heart, so is he.

When a sick person constantly convinces himself that he will never get well, it becomes almost certain that his negativity and troubles will carry him to the grave.

Flesh is dumb! We never want you to forget that statement. That is the reason we use it over and over again. The mind, your human computer, is really the controlling factor in your entire body makeup. Flesh cannot think for itself because only the mind does the thinking. That is why you must cultivate strong, healthy Positive Thinking.

Your Mind Must Control Your Body!

The mind must have a will of iron and always be in command of the body. From this day forward learn how to substitute thoughts. When a negative thought – such as, *"I am losing my energy because when you get older you start to lose energy"* – enters your mind, replace it with positive thoughts, say, *"Age cannot in any way affect my energy. Age is not toxic! I am ageless!"*

Keep in mind always that whatever the mind tells the flesh, that is exactly what the flesh is going to believe and act upon. Your mind influences flesh. You must let your mind make decisions for your body, because if your body rules your mind, you face a life of misery and slavery!

Are You Poisoning Your Body?

If you are eating the kind of food most Americans and people of other affluent industrialized countries eat, you are slowly poisoning yourself and dulling your brain. You are filling yourself with *foodless* foods and depriving your body of natural nutrition it needs. You may also be among many who hasten this suicidal process by adding toxic poisons: tobacco, alcohol, coffee, caffeine teas, soda and cola drinks.

There is a great deal of discussion in the media today about polluted air and water. What about a polluted bloodstream? Here is something you can do: Start today to detoxify your entire body and rebuild and revitalize it with healthy organic foods and healthy lifestyle living!

A Healthy Mind for Health and Long Life

What has your mind to do with health and long life? Far more than the majority of men and women realize! Think of your thoughts as powerful self-talk magnets with the ability to attract (positive) or repel (negative) according to the way used. A majority of people lean either to positive or negative side mentally. The positive phase is constructive and goes for success and positive achievements, while the negative side of life is destructive, leading to futility and failure. It's self-evident it's to our advantage to cultivate a positive, healthy, mental attitude. With patience, persistence and living The Bragg Healthy Lifestyle this can be accomplished!

There are many negative and destructive forms of thought which react in every cell in your body. The strongest is fear, and its child, worry – along with depression, anxiety, apprehension, jealousy, ill-will, envy, anger, resentment, vengefulness and self-pity. All of these negative thoughts bring tension to the body and mind, leading to waste of energy, enervation and also slow or rapid poisoning of the body. Rage, intense fear and shock are very violent and quickly intoxicate the whole system. Worry and other destructive emotions act slowly but, in the end, have the same destructive effect. Anger and intense fear stop digestive action, upset the kidneys and the colon causing total body upheaval (diarrhea or constipation, headaches, pains, fever, etc.).

Fear, worry and other destructive habits of thought muddle the mind! A crystal clear mind is needed to reason to your best advantage, enabling you to make sound, healthy decisions. An emotionally, upset clouded mind often makes unwise and unhealthy decisions and might be unable to reach any positive conclusions at all!

What are positive, healthy, mental forces or expressions? They are the ones that lead to peace of mind and inner relaxation, as opposed to the destructive habits which cause a tightening-up of the entire body system. This very second, relax, let your positive mind take over your body!

Who is strong? He that can conquer his bad habits. – Ben Franklin

Leaving positive, encouraging, kind messages on Post-It notes for others, even strangers can sparkle and change a life! – See web: OperationBeautiful.com

Anger & Hostility – Big Heart Disease Risks

New studies from John Hopkins School of Medicine and University of Maryland have found that irritability, hostility and dominance may cause coronary heart disease. Until recently, most research centered on the role of psychosocial factors, says Dr. Aron Siegman. The study involved 101 men and 95 women, the average age was 55 years. The research found that a full-blown outward expression of anger is a risk factor for coronary heart disease in men, and for women – subtle, indirect expressions of antagonism and anger are big risk factors! Also, expressions of irritability with anger are risk factors for coronary heart disease. (See web: *drsinatra.com*)

Death rates from heart disease are up 4 to 7 times higher among people with hostile, mean attitudes, stated by Dr. Redford Williams, Duke University Medical Center. Read his book *Anger Kills* available through *Amazon.com*

Drugs Control Addict's Mind!

The *drug addict* is the extreme example of the body ruling the mind! This is why the world is over-populated with drug addicts. The body's craving forces the mind to command the body to commit violent crimes for money needed to buy the drugs it craves! Sadly, this is why the world is becoming crime riddled by drug addicts!

We maintain most bad habits simply because our minds are enslaved by our bodies. This applies to alcohol, coffee, caffeine teas and other stimulants. The body rules by the false philosophy of *"Eat, drink and be merry, for tomorrow we die."* This is false. You don't die tomorrow, but if you continue to live by this wrong philosophy, 5, 10, 20 years later you could be burdened with a sick, prematurely aged body tormenting you daily!

A Harvard Study show men with highest anger on personality tests are three times more likely to develop heart disease. High blood pressure affects 1 in 3 of all adults in the U.S.; it is often called "the silent killer".

In the Framingham Heart Study, women who reported suppressing their anger experienced the highest rate of first heart attacks.

Stress puts an unhealthy strain on the heart. A UCLA study found 6 out of 10 heart patients had constricted arteries and reduced blood flow to their heart following any emotionally charged upsets or events.

Exercise, yoga, prayer, cheerfulness, smile, relax & heal. – Patricia Bragg, ND, PhD.

Chapter 8

Doctor Deep Breathing

When You Breathe Deeply and Fully You Live Healthier and Longer

When you pump a generous flow of oxygen into your body, 100 trillion cells become more alive! This enables the four main *motors* of your body – the heart, lungs, liver and kidneys – to operate and perform better. Your miracle-working bloodstream purifies and cleanses every part of the body, including itself. This eliminates toxic wastes as Mother Nature planned, and the fuel (food) and vital oxygen are carried to every cell in your body.

With ample oxygen your muscles, tendons and joints function more smoothly. Your skin becomes firmer and more resilient and your complexion clearer and more glowing. You will then radiate with greater health and well-being for a longer, healthier life!

With the Bragg Super Power Breathing your brain becomes more alert and your nervous system functions better. You become free from tension and strain because you can easily take the stresses and pressures of daily living. Your emotions come under control. You feel joyous and exuberant. If negative emotions such as anger, hate, jealousy, greed or fear intrude, you can expel them by positive thinking and slow, concentrated deep breathing.

The deep breather enjoys more peace of mind, tranquility and serenity. In India, the great teachers practice deep, full breathing as the first essential step towards higher spiritual development. You can attain higher concentration in prayers and meditation by taking long, slow, deep breaths. Also, deep breathing stimulates your brain cells and promotes new brain cell growth.

On an average day your lungs move enough air in and out to fill a medium-sized room or blow up several thousand party balloons.

Oxygen is the vital, precious, invisible staff of life. – Paul C. Bragg, ND, PhD.

Just by paying attention to breathing, you can access new levels of health and relaxation that will benefit every area of your life. – Deepak Chopra, M.D.

The quality of breath should be deep, graceful, easy and efficient. – Kenneth Cohen, Health Educator

Super Deep Breathing Improves Brain Power

The person who breathes deeply and fully thinks more clearly and sharply. Oxygen stimulates your brain and logic and intelligence. The more deeply and fully you breathe, the greater your power of concentration and the more your creative mind asserts itself. You will also develop greater extrasensory perception within your body, especially the brain. Scientists at the Salk Institute for Biological Studies, La Jolla, CA, now know adults do generate new brain cells in the hippocampus, an area in the brain which is responsible for learning and memory. Deep breathing nourishes and fine-tunes the brain and entire body! (*salk.edu*)

Do read *Bragg Super Power Breathing* book (page 251) for it shows how to enjoy high energy vibration living! The more fully and deeply you breathe, the further you will travel to higher levels on the physical, mental and spiritual planes. Now close your eyes. Relax a few minutes while doing some slow, deep breathing! See web: *bragg.com* for some relaxing breathing techniques.

The Lungs Are Nature's Miracle Breathers

Every animal extracts oxygen from the environment in which it lives. Through their gills, fish extract oxygen from water. Insects get oxygen from the air through alveoli, or air cells, in individual openings set in segments of their bodies. Worms and other invertebrates breathe through the pores of their skin. Vertebrate animals, including the human race, have those miracle mechanisms – the lungs. The mechanical equivalent would be a pair of bellows, though the lungs are far more intricate and adaptable. Human lungs are a miracle pair of conical-shaped organs composed of spongy, porous tissue. They occupy the thoracic cavity (chest) with the heart in the center, and are protected by the amazingly strong and resilient rib cage. The apex of each lung reaches just above the collar bone; the base extends to the waistline.

What makes up our lungs? About 800 million alveoli – air cells or sacs of elastic tissue – which can expand or contract like tiny balloons. If these little air sacs were flattened out and laid side by side, the flattened alveoli would cover an area of 100 square yards!

Tiny capillaries (blood vessels) thread the elastic lung walls of each of the millions of air sacs . . . and it is through these that the blood passes to discharge its load of poisonous carbon dioxide and absorb the vital, life-giving oxygen. The average person has five to six quarts of blood, which must be cleansed continually.

Air inhaled through the nose and mouth reaches the alveoli through an intricate system of tubes, beginning with the large trachea, or windpipe, which is kept rigid by rings of cartilage in its walls. The trachea extends through the neck into the chest, where it divides into two branches (bronchi), each leading into a lung cavity. Each bronchus divides into a number of successively smaller branches to bring air to every air sac.

You Have Lungs – Fill Them Up

Each lung sits perfectly enveloped in a protective elastic membrane, the pleura, whose inner layer is attached to the lung, and it's outer layer forms the lining of the thoracic cavity inside the rib cage. One end of each rib is attached to the spinal column, but the front of the rib cage is open. This allows the lungs to expand and contract. When you breathe deeply, filling every air sac, your thoracic cavity expands as your lungs fill with six to ten pints of air. This varies according to body build and size. Lungs occupy from 200 to over 300 cubic inches.

This marvelous breathing mechanism is yours for free! You are born with it. It functions without conscious effort, yet without it, you can't exist. Not even the latest inventions used by hospitals in emergencies, however ingenious, can equal the human breathing apparatus. Perhaps if human beings had to pay a fabulous price for their lungs and air, they would use them to full capacity all the time. Think of the big price you pay for only using them partially by shallow breathing. Remember, we are always only one breath away from death! **Now, start enjoying slow, deep relaxed breathing and feel how your body responds.**

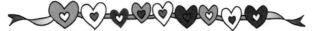

I have shared the Bragg Super Power Breathing with thousands at my Sports Seminars around the world. It creates champions – it super-charges your life!
– Bob Anderson, World Famous Stretching Coach (www.stretching.com)

The Importance of Clean Air to Health

It is essential to breathe clean air – air that's as free as possible from such chemicals as smog, car exhaust, natural gas appliance fumes and the many other toxic chemical pollutants. Also, our air needs to be as free as possible from mold, dust, dust mites and their fecal matter, animal dander and pollen. Everyone's health is helped in varying degrees by clean air. It is vitally important to live and work in an area which has clean air and which is free of all harmful fumes. It is also equally important to keep our homes pure, clean and free from dust, dust mites and debris! Most people cannot be truly 100% healthy and well until they breathe clean air, maintain a healthy diet and live a healthy lifestyle.

Pollutants Threaten the Lungs of All Life

Every living thing breathes. In the marvelous balance of Mother Nature, plants breathe in carbon dioxide through the pores in their leaves and give off vital oxygen – while animals inhale oxygen and exhale carbon dioxide. Both thrive in a healthy, natural balance.

70

Unfortunately, humans have played havoc with this natural balance by destroying forests and covering grass with pavement. They continue to poison our already over-burdened air with pollutants from motorized traffic and heavy industry. Wildlife, when it survives slaughter by humanity, suffocates in such polluted air. Fish die in polluted waters. How long can people survive in the midst of these environmental poisons which they continually create? This is a question of great concern to us. Read the classic book *Silent Spring* by our friend Rachel Carson, available in most libraries. If followed, her wise advice would have saved America and other nations billions of dollars and countless wildlife species! We desperately need more courageous and dedicated people like Rachel Carson to show the world the error of its poisonous, killing ways!

Airplanes are spraying chemicals across our skies that are on OSHA hazardous list. Chemtrails have returned positive for toxic aluminum, barium, bacteria, virus and molds, causing health problems. Check web: chemtrails911.com

Your breathing habits are the first place, not the last, one should look when fatigue, disease or other evidence of disordered energy presents itself.
– Dr. Sheldon Hendler, *The Oxygen Breakthrough* (Amazon.com)

Live Longer Breathing Clean Air Deeply

We advise those who have to live or work in smoggy, polluted cities to obtain a good air filter. We especially recommend filters which contain charcoal and a high efficiency particulate HEPA air filter. The charcoal removes most of the chemicals and the HEPA filter removes most of the particles. To be effective in an average room, the flow rate through the filter should be over 200 cubic feet of air per minute. The wise motorist will also install an air filter in his car for cleaning the air while driving in air-polluted cities. Auto stores and catalogs usually stock them.

When we are born, our lungs are new, fresh, clean, and rosy in color. If we could live in a pollutant and dust-free atmosphere breathing deeply all our lives, then our lungs would remain *as good as new* for a long life of use. Yet most people abuse their lungs! Some of this comes from external causes. The lungs and skin are the only organs of the body which are directly affected by external conditions, specifically, the air breathed into the lungs!

Mother Nature and God provide protection against normal amount of dust contamination: tiny nose hairs serve as filters, and moist mucus in passages leading to lungs traps dust particles that we expel through the nose or mouth. The tonsils also serve as important guards to trap germs. The lungs protect themselves remarkably well by expelling carbon dioxide through oxygenation and by discharging toxins into the blood for elimination via kidneys. *Your body is a miracle!*

Unfortunately, most civilized people today live in very unnatural conditions. Almost everywhere there are abnormal pollutants in the air we breathe, especially in urban areas. Our lungs are often overloaded with more contaminants than they can handle. These are passed into the bloodstream and to other parts of the body. Modern city dweller's lungs become brownish from car smog, soot, etc. Even in most farming areas, the lungs must contend with pollens, excessive dust, poisonous pesticides, fertilizers and other toxic chemicals. (Air purifiers and vitamin C helps.)

SHOCKING DEADLY FACT: *Smog kills over 300 people yearly in #1 smog-riddled Los Angeles. This study has also estimated that this figure could triple soon! Please read our* Bragg Super Power Breathing Book.

Tobacco – Enemy of Your Heart and Health

Whether it's cigarettes, cigars or pipes, tobacco is one of the heart's worst enemies! Here is what Dr. Lester M. Morrison, noted California heart specialist and pioneer in the low-cholesterol diet for the treatment and the prevention of heart disease, said about tobacco:

Tobacco is a poison. Nicotine, the main ingredient of tobacco, is a poison affecting the brain, heart and other vital organs. The tobacco plant is directly related to the deadly nightshade family of plants. Aside from the chief poison, nicotine, there are other well-known poisons present in tobacco: arsenic and coal tar substances and the carbon monoxide when tobacco is burned. See smoking facts page 75.

Dr. Morrison also said, *Nicotine is the most noxious substance that affects the blood vessels in man. Nicotine is a powerful drug that constricts the arteries, narrowing still more the vital passageways of the blood, already clogged by other toxic residue. The tobacco smoker does double damage to his heart – first, by filling the bloodstream with the harsh poisons of tobacco and, second, by narrowing the arteries and other blood vessels, preventing a free flow of life-giving blood.*

72

Smoking Has Many Ways to Kill You!

The body has no defense against carbon monoxide produced by smoking. You have read about people committing suicide or being killed by carbon monoxide fumes. Why deliberately breathe fumes into your lungs? The coal tars in tobacco are the chief poisons responsible for cancer of the lungs, mouth and related areas of the body. It frightens us to think of what will happen in another 25 years because of the excessive use of tobacco. We are convinced that every smoker (marijuana also) will develop **lung, throat or some form of cancer,** if **heart disease** or something else doesn't kill them first!

The results of a recent federal health study found that cigars are no less hazardous than other forms of tobacco, and therefore needs stronger federal regulation! The absence of such warning labels on cigars could lead consumers to erroneously conclude cigars don't carry health risks. Beware, there is no safe form of deadly tobacco!

Cigars are becoming more popular and sales have jumped way up. Yet cigar smokers and tobacco chewers face grave risk of many diseases as cancer in mouth, throat, esophageal, larynx and lung cancer, as well as coronary heart disease and chronic obstructive pulmonary disease. Fact: cigars contain up to 90 times as much of the cancer-causing agents as cigarettes do!

Emphysema Smothers it's Victim

Emphysema, another killer disease from smoking, is on the rise. Recent medical reports show that as many as half of all American men are suffering from some degree of emphysema. In this disease, the tars, nicotine and other destructive poisons of tobacco lodge in the lungs' small air sacs, causing the sac walls to become very thin or to break down entirely. Soon the blood is no longer able to exchange poisonous carbon dioxide for life-giving oxygen. This self-destructing victim dies of oxygen starvation – being slowly smothered to death from within.

Emphysema is not a quick killer. It creeps up slowly, first with a slight cough – especially on arising. Then it attacks the smoker day and night. Slowly, air sacs are almost completely destroyed. The victim doesn't die suddenly, but lingers on steadily deteriorating. They are forced to stay near an oxygen tank because the disease is shutting off their oxygen. When the lungs can't operate any longer even with pure oxygen, the victim then dies.

Our breath is our life! We can live days without water and weeks without food, but only minutes without air. It's the oxygen in the air we breathe that's the greatest purifying force in Mother Nature! To get this oxygen into the lungs and bloodstream, we must breathe it in!

Smoking tobacco is against every Natural Law. When you attempt to break a Law of Mother Nature, it will soon break you! *The heart needs large oxygen amounts to function.* Any disease that diminishes oxygen is going to destroy the health of your heart, lungs and entire body!

The study showed most heavy smokers are snorers and are at a 1.7 times greater risk of heart disease than silent sleepers and at 2.08 times greater risk of stroke and heart disease combined. – Finnish Medical Study

Vitamin C Protects Heart, Arteries & Body

Vitamin C is one of Mother Nature's most essential elements for good health. In addition to its other vital functions – such as prevention of scurvy, vitamin C is also active in preventing capillaries hemorrhaging, those tiny blood vessels that directly feed the body's cells. (We take 1,000 to 3,000 mg mixed "C" daily, plus grapeseed extract.)

Smoking Robs Your Body of Vitamin C

Tobacco neutralizes Vitamin C in your body, robbing you of its vital protection. Dr. W. J. McCormick – Canada's "C" Specialist – found in lab and clinical tests *smoking of a single cigarette robs body of the amount of vitamin C contained in 1 medium sized orange.* A *pack a day* smoker would have to eat 20 oranges for enough "C" in his body! Tobacco is not the only "C" thief, polluted air and foods with preservatives are also.

When capillaries in the artery walls hemorrhage, there is additional blockage to the blood flow. When this occurs in the heart or brain, a serious clot may form. In the legs and feet serious breakdown of the capillaries may occur. Sometimes this leads to gangrene, requiring an amputation and sometimes it causes varicose veins. So you can see how essential Vitamin C is to the healthy functioning of your heart, bloodstream and entire body.

All Smokers – Stop Smoking Today!

Many smokers are so addicted to this unhealthy and filthy habit that they become cry babies, saying, *"It's impossible for me to break the habit of smoking."* All we can say is, Rubbish! *Who controls your body – the tobacco or you?* Flesh is dumb! It has no intelligence. Your mind (your miracle computer) must control your body! The mind can always force the body to obey its orders!

QUIT SMOKING! All smokers must stop this vicious, deadly habit that destroys health, youth, energy and life!
See web: cdc.gov/tobacco

It doesn't matter how much or how long you've been smoking — stop now and in one year your risk of heart disease will be cut by 70%.
– Dr. Daniel Levy, *Framingham Heart Study Director*

DEADLY SMOKING FACTS!

✝ Tobacco use and second-hand smoke will eventually kill 1/5 of developed world population: about 250 million people.

✝ Of the 50 million Americans who smoke, one third to one half will die from a smoke-related disease. All will reduce their life expectancy by an average of nine years.

✝ Smoking acts as either a stimulant or a depressant, depending upon the smoker's emotional state.

✝ The average pack-a-day smoker takes about 70,000 hits of nicotine each year and with 2 packs it's 140,000 hits.

✝ "Second hand smoke" hurts non-smokers: it speeds up the heart rate, raises blood pressure and doubles the amount of deadly carbon monoxide in their blood.

✝ Secondary smoke contains more nicotine, cadmium and tar than mainstream smoke. It leads to hypertension, bronchitis, asthma and deadly emphysema.

✝ Babies born to mothers who smoke tend to not be as healthy, have lower body weight and smaller lungs.

✝ Lung illnesses are twice as common in smokers' children.

75

✝ Children and teenagers make up 90% of the new smokers in the United States – and teenage smoking is on the rise!

✝ Death rate from heart disease and breast cancer ranges from 25% to 75% higher among women who smoke.

✝ Female smokers may face a higher risk of lung cancer – as much as twice the risk of male smokers, according to Dr. Harvey Risch's study at Yale University.

✝ Your body contains over 60,000 miles of blood vessels. Smoking constricts those vessels, causing heart trouble and depriving your body of fresh, rich oxygen it needs.

✝ Tobacco is the main introduction to more deadly drugs.

✝ Teens who smoke are far more likely to engage in other risky and life-threatening behaviors than non-smoking teens (including using other dangerous drugs, violence, gang involvement, carrying weapons, and engaging in premarital sex, which often results in pregnancy or disease).

✝ Cataracts, cancer, angina, heart disease, osteoporosis, bronchitis, high blood pressure, impotency, diabetes asthma and respiratory ailments are linked to smoking.

A Deep Desire Has Great Power

In our Bragg Health Crusades worldwide we have had health *students in our classes who have smoked for as many as 60 years – and they stopped, without tapering off.* They simply made up their minds to stop smoking at once – and they did. They stopped without the use of nicotine patches, nicotine gum, etc., as these are dangerous too!

Of course the brave souls who are quitting suffer for a few days as their nerves cry out for the nicotine *fix* of the deadly tobacco. However, they find the intestinal fortitude and purpose to take the brief punishment of their withdrawal discomforts. They are fighting a monster that controlled them. They can and will win their battle!

To be effective in changing a bad habit into a good one, rational thought must be accompanied by deep feeling and desire. If you desire a Healthy Heart strongly enough, you can and will conquer the tobacco habit!

Picture yourself as you would like to be. Believe for the moment that such an image is possible. In forming good habits and breaking bad ones, we have to deal with *thought habits. As a man thinketh in his heart, so is he.* Think, *No smoking!* Tell yourself over and over that smoking is a deadly habit, it is slowly killing you and that it's your enemy! Say to yourself over and over again, *Tobacco in any form is a killer and I am through with this vicious poison forever!* Repeat, *I will not smoke!* over and over again. You will soon become master of your body, instead of a slave to the tobacco (and marijuana) habit!

76

It's Up To You To Be Happier and Healthier!

Actions speak louder than words and can elevate your mood if you feel depressed. Take a walk and do slow, deep breathing – it helps you sort out and solve problems. Spend time with children – it simplifies life and puts everything in perspective. Find the comics or something funny to read and laugh about. If someone is upset, try to analyze the situation from that person's perspective. Make yourself physically smile and laugh; it opens blood vessels in the back of your head to physically lift your mood. Choose to be happy in spite of circumstances. No one "makes" you happy – it's an attitude you self-create from within. – *Paul C. Bragg*

Chapter 9

Doctor Exercise

Mind over Muscle

The saying, *If you don't use it, you lose it,* certainly applies to the 640 muscles of the human body. When you don't exercise regularly, your muscles lose their firm, supple tone. Over time they can become soft and flabby.

If overweight, make up your mind that you want to trim down to your normal weight. This is more difficult than it seems, because the mind has a way of making excuses for an overweight body. For instance, you may say to yourself, *It's normal for me to be fat. I'm the plump type,* or, *I eat so little, yet I remain fat.* The latter may be true – remember it is what you eat, not how much! And it is never normal to be obese and over-fuel your body!

Your mind must control your body! Flesh is dumb and flesh is weak. Flesh often demands fatty, starchy, sugary foods. Either your mind rules the body or the body rules the mind. Be positive! Tell your body that your mind is going to be your health captain and wisely guide you! 77

Exercise Daily for a Powerful Heart

Remember that it is a lean horse that finishes the long race! If you want a long, healthy life, keep your body trim and fit. Once you have trimmed down to your normal weight through proper diet and daily exercise, there will be a huge difference in the way you will feel! You will be bubbling over with vitality and energy. You will be unafraid of life's challenges and be free from the fear of heart trouble and other illnesses!

Laziness is a vicious habit. Sitting too much can ruin your health and is a bad habit. You need to devote *1 to 2 hours daily* to a variety of exercise, gardening, etc. The simplest and best is brisk walking for a strong heart, preferably up and down hills, or even walking up and down steps.

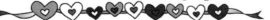

Regular exercise is a critical part of staying healthy. There are 1,440 minutes in every day. Schedule 30 of them for physical activity! – nlm.nih.gov/hinfo.html

Duty is a matter of the mind. Dedication is a matter of the heart.

Enjoy Exercising – It's Healthy and Fun!

There is great hiking near where we had a home in Hollywood, California, where Mt. Hollywood rises some 2,000 feet in famous Griffith Park. We enjoyed early morning hikes up the mountain to greet the sun rising and then run down. Also, in Santa Barbara, we always enjoy ocean swimming and hiking the surrounding hills.

We love to walk, jog and climb mountains. We take time to walk or jog daily, or we swim, play tennis or ride our bikes. We work out 3 times a week with a progressive weight training program, which helps keep our bones and muscles healthier and stronger. See pages 95 to 96.

Exercise is the greatest single factor available to us for removing any blockages and unclogging the arteries and blood vessels, and for increasing the vital flow of oxygen-enriched blood throughout the heart and body. Recent studies show that exercise can reduce the risk of developing adult-onset diabetes as well as breast cancer. The famous Harvard School of Public Health Researchers (*www.health.harvard.edu*) studied a group of 70,000 women. Results: 46% lowered their risk of diabetes with daily vigorous exercising and brisk walking.

78

Your Heart Muscle – Thrives on Exercise

Your heart is a muscle and muscles need and thrive on ample exercise! Challenging the heart through aerobic exercises such as brisk walking, running, bicycling or swimming helps it to beat more efficiently. Exercise actually expands the blood vessels around the heart, which can be a lifesaver if a blood clot latches onto one of your coronary arteries.

According to Dr. Pamela Peeke, author of *Fit to Live*, "An out-of-shape heart can be hazardous. Fat infiltrates the heart muscle and can interfere with electrical impulses. This may cause arrhythmia, or even sudden death." (*amazon.com*)

American Heart Association states that exercise is especially important for those with heart disease. They recommend that you first undergo a stress test; utilizing a heart rate monitor while you work-out is helpful. See web: *aarpmagazine.org*.

Only 20% of American's have some form of regular exercise! This is causing poor health and more cardiovascular disease! Regular exercise is important for your Bragg Healthy Heart Program. Please start your exercise program today.

Develop Strength from the Inside Out, Not from the Outside In

Remember that from the day you were born into this world, to the day you die, your 640 muscles play an important role in everything you do. Think of it – *more than half of your body is sheer active, working muscle!* It isn't the muscles that you see that count as much as those you don't see! Along the 30-foot gastrointestinal tract there are muscles to force food along this tube. The work of bringing adequate amounts of air into your powerful lungs also requires other strong muscles.

And above all, *the greatest muscle* in your body is *your heart, your number one pump.* It is the heart that pumps the blood supply into the body's 640 muscles. And the more we bring these 640 muscles into play, the better our heart, circulation, physical condition and our entire state of health will be! You have four more extra *pumps* that can also help this whole miracle process – they are your two arms and your two legs – use and exercise them!

Brisk Power Walking is the King of Exercise

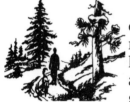 Brisk power walking is the best form of aerobic exercise because it brings most of the body into action which helps open up blocked blood vessels and builds your endurance. Your heart grows in strength and efficiency, able to function with less strain. Also, many problems and upsets get solved on walks. As you walk, grasp yourself in small of back *(press knuckles 3 minute sessions into any back pains)*. Your entire frame responds to every step. Feel how chief muscles function rhythmically. No other exercise gives the same harmony of coordinating sinews and same perfect circulation of blood. Brisk power walking is ideal for you, your health and your heart! (We also enjoy ocean swimming.)

You have to eat healthy to treat your arteries and heart well. If you don't challenge your body by working it through exercise, brisk walking, etc. your heart muscle and your entire cardiovascular system will not work at their best.

The goal of exercise & weight loss should be to reduce any abdominal fat deposits that will help lower potential for cardiovascular disease (page 57).

Exercise, along with some fasting helps maintain and restore a healthy, physical balance and normal weight for a long, happy life. – Paul C. Bragg

Walk 2 to 3 Miles Daily – It Does Miracles!
Get Fit – Firm up – Lose Fat – De-stress

You should try to walk 2-3 miles daily, and some times try doubling it. Don't give yourself excuses. *Make a daily walk a permanent part of your Bragg Healthy Heart Fitness Program* – all year and in all climates. Conrad Hilton walked in the sun, also rain and loved it (page 52). Regardless what other exercises you do, your daily walk is a *must*! Of course, you may take it in the form of golf if you enjoy this social sport. But it's best not to ride around the golf course in an electric cart! This makes a farce of the whole thing. Walking is what your heart needs. We are inclined to agree with Mark Twain, who said, *Golf is a good way to spoil a good walk.* But, if it takes the game to make you walk, do so. The result is almost the same – healthy functioning muscles and quickened blood circulation, plus a sense of harmony and happiness!

Although the outdoors is preferable – where you can get the most fresh air – indoor walking is far better than none at all. In winter, you can try hallways, porches or shopping malls. When on health crusades around the world, we take an evening brisk walk through the corridors, and up and down the stairs of our hotel. If a roof terrace is available, we prefer this open-air space.

80

Expert Advice on How to Exercise

Often you may ask yourself, "Why aren't you closing in on your ideal weight?" You're trying to workout and exercise, but it doesn't seem your bathroom scale is showing you any results – your weight appears the same as when you started out. Here are some tips from the exercise experts:

- An effective weekly exercise program to get your heart in shape should include one rigorous program that makes you sweat; two moderate exercise programs, and one easy session. For example: taking an aerobics class, or a run and after a more relaxing yoga or stretching class.

- Drink at least 8 glasses of distilled, purified or reverse osmosis water daily. Drinking water has a huge effect on exercise. Dehydrated exercisers worked out 25% less than those who drank water before, during and after exercise.

London Bus Conductors who walked up and down the stairs of their double-decker buses had a lower rate of heart disease deaths than the London Bus Drivers who sat all day driving the bus.

• In initial phases of exercise training, you may get a post-workout drop in blood sugar that causes cravings for simple carbohydrates like sweets. However, cravings should disappear a few weeks into your exercise training. Have delicious fresh fruits handy such as organic apples, oranges, pears and bananas, rather than reaching for an unhealthy chocolate bar or soft drink filled with sugar. Instead enjoy Bragg Healthy Organic Vinegar Drinks (see page 256).

To Enjoy Your Daily Walk Is Important

Your walking should never be done self-consciously, no heel and toe routine and no time limiting. Let it be the most functional and enjoyable of exercises. Walk naturally – with head high, spine stretched up, chest out, tummy in. Swing hips, arms and body into action. Walk as though legs began at the middle of torso. Breathe deeply! You will feel physical elation and will carry yourself proudly with body erect and arms swinging easily from shoulders. Move at your own pace, with a free spirit and a light heart. If you want, listen to motivational tapes or music. As you walk, your body ceases to matter, you become as near a poet and nature philosopher as you will ever be.

81

Walk your worries away! As blood courses through your arteries and veins, cleansing and nourishing your body, you are filled with a sense of well-being that clears your mind of troubles and nourishes it with healthy positive thoughts. As Dad and I stride along on our hikes, we say to ourselves and sometimes aloud with each step – *Health! Strength! Youth! Vitality! Love! for Eternity!*

It's beneficial to also take a hiking tour once a year. Select interesting areas which you, your family and friends would like to see, and hike about 15 miles daily. You will broaden your knowledge of our beautiful planet and of Mother Nature, as well as help to build a more powerful, healthier and long-lasting heart. The websites listed below will help you in your selection.

Websites to inspire you into healthy walking, jogging & hiking

- *www.walking.about.com*
- *www.apma.org/sports/walking*
- *www.mayoclinic.com/health/walking*
- *www.TheWalkingSite.com*
- *www.aarp.org/walking*
- *www.SierraClub.com*

Walking – Running – Perfect Conditioners

We love jogging and walking – because a *run a day helps keep heart attacks away!* We also enjoy light jogging, as practiced by athletes in training workouts. Do this with an easy sustained pace, head up, shoulders back, arms swinging naturally. All athletes and trainers worldwide consider running and jogging as perfect conditioners.

Enjoy Exercise & Jogs for Longer Life

On our world Bragg Health Crusades the first question we ask the hotel manager is, *Where is the nearest park where we can take our daily exercise?* And off we go sometime during the day. We prefer to go early in the morning or late in the afternoon. Each person, however, should choose the time best suited and available to them.

We are so pleased to find that all over the world today running and jogging have become an accepted method in the pursuit of Heart Fitness by people of all age groups. Many cities have hiking and jogging clubs, which anyone may join. We have had the pleasure of running with folks everywhere we go: including Europe, England, Australia, New Zealand, Asia and throughout the world and U.S.

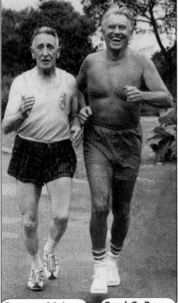

Duncan McLean · Paul C. Bragg

It is universally accepted that exercise is important for the promotion of physical, mental and emotional health. A daily run, jog or fast walk – when adapted to your physical and mental condition and age – will strongly improve endurance, produce a sense of well-being and help maintain total body fitness (plus each step gives your trillions of cells a massage and trampolining does also). Exercise helps increase resistance to sickness and disease, and helps make the heart healthier, fit, stronger and last longer!

Paul Bragg with friend Duncan McLean, England's oldest Champion Sprinter, (83 years young) on a training run in London's beautiful Regent's Park.

Before starting on your exercise program, it's wise to seek advice from your health practitioner. Also, be sure that you choose a soft surface to run or jog on, such as grass or sand. Jogging on hard surfaces, such as concrete and asphalt, could accumulate damage to knees, hips, ankles and organs.

Exercise is the Best Fitness Conditioner

A daily program of walking, running or jogging is a quick, sure and inexpensive fitness conditioner. Be faithful to your exercise routine for true heart fitness. Women will be especially pleased when they see fat change to lean, as the inches fly off their waistlines and hiplines – all the while improving their health! Men and women, both please remember your waistline is your lifeline and also your dateline! A person with a trim and fit figure always looks more youthful and attractive!

If you are a *softie* and feel you cannot get outside for your run or jog on cold and rainy days – stationary inside jogging to music or your favorite talk show will work too. Stay in one place and lift one foot at a time about 6-8 inches from floor – it's best to start easy and gradually build up to faster, longer periods. Remember to exercise where you get the most fresh air – on the patio, front porch, or inside or outside rest areas at work. 83

The Miracle Life of Ageless Jack LaLanne

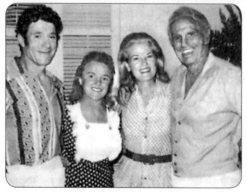

Jack LaLanne, Patricia Bragg, Elaine LaLanne & Paul C. Bragg

Jack says he would have been dead by 16 if he hadn't attended The Bragg Crusade. Jack says, *Bragg saved my life at age 15, when I attended the Bragg Health and Fitness Crusade in Oakland, California.* From that day, Jack has continued to live The Bragg Healthy Lifestyle, inspiring millions to health, fitness and a long fulfilled, happy life!

See Jack LaLanne's website: *www.jacklalanne.com*

Exercising in the Sky – You Arrive Healthier

We even get our jogging in while thousands of feet high in the air, soaring the skies in a airplane. We just go to the rear of the plane and jog and stretch. We never arrive stiff and tired. Learn to take advantage of any spare moments for stationary jogging during the day, whether you are an office worker, CEO or housewife. We all must have daily exercise for good, healthy hearts and bodies.

Good Shoes & Socks Promote Happy Feet

Comfortable walking shoes with flexible rubber soles under the heels is important. We often insert foam inner soles, Dr. Scholl's – our friend and follower who said Bragg Foot Book is "Best Foot Program Ever!". Safeguard your precious feet with good serviceable shoes and ample padding! Otherwise, the continual hard jarring of walking, jogging and exercising in ill-fitting or thin-soled shoes can eventually cause some foot discomfort and discouragement! Shoes should not be too loose or overly tight. Feet often swell from added stimulation and circulation caused by running and when shoes are too tight you can get painful blisters! Your socks must fit right. Make sure they haven't any holes or repairs that could cause chafing or blistering. Be sure your socks aren't the kind that bunch up inside your shoes. For sports we often wear 2 pairs of socks – first a thin cotton pair, then a heavier wool – just as many tennis champs do.

Try and *do your jogging on grass or soft surfaces*. Grass is easier on the legs and feet, especially if you are a big person. Your legs carry you throughout life and deserve every consideration you can give them! In addition to comfortable clothes and a good exercise space, you will need willpower and a dedicated purpose to keep at it! When first starting you might be hindered by unaccustomed aches, pains and blisters. Remember, this needed soreness is often a healthy sign that important fitness changes are underway in your body. Think of any temporary discomfort in this way and you'll even take pride in feeling stiff for a few days. Take a hot apple cider vinegar bath (add 1/2 cup apple cider vinegar). The big rule to follow is: *train, but don't overdo and strain*!

Alternate Running and Walking
"One step begins a ten thousand mile journey."

A wise Chinese proverb to start your new, exciting journey toward Healthy Heart Fitness with a winning attitude! One yard is approximately the longest step you can take. Now, step off 25 yards or 50, 75 or 100 and slowly increase the distance and do more sets. Initially run any of these distances. If you have not been exercising, make your first weeks' daily runs 25-50 yards. Run or jog whatever distance you choose as a starter. After the run, then walk the same distance, briskly and breathe deeply while keeping your head and shoulders up and your arms swinging. Deep breathing is important. The reason you are doing this exercise is to give your heart more oxygen. Dad and I are faithful to our fast walking/running program. Walking/running every day helps your heart get stronger!

Daily Walk and Run Brings Miracles

When you walk and run daily, the sustained pressure on the circulatory system adds elasticity to the blood vessels, increasing their capacity for greater and easier blood flow. It's remarkable that this simple exercise can be such a positive step in protecting your heart and health. A great Heart Specialist in London told us that any person who runs 15-30 minutes daily for a year could expect to double the capacity of their main arteries. *This is the way to build a powerful heart.* Activity (brisk walking, jogging, running, etc.) that causes deep breathing requires more energy. The body produces this energy by burning foodstuffs – the burning agent is oxygen. The body can store food at each meal, using what it wants and saving the rest for later, but it can't store oxygen. Most of us produce enough energy to perform ordinary daily activities. But as physical activity becomes more vigorous, the unfit just can't keep up, because the means for oxygen delivery is limited in their bodies. This is what separates the fit from the unfit!

You can dramatically lower your risk of dying prematurely simply by walking briskly or engaging in other aerobic activities on a regular basis. You will lower your blood pressure and blood cholesterol, control your weight, improve your quality of life and get better quality sleep.

To find a suitable pulmonary rehabilitation exercise program ask your doctor or investigate what's offered at your local hospitals or YMCA.

> **Like a car, regular maintenance and sensible use can keep the human miracle heart working in an *as new* condition even at a vintage age! – Paul Bragg, ND, PhD.**

Jogging and running demands you to breathe more oxygen in and forces your body to process and deliver it. Even if you have been inactive or sick, start simple walking and light exercise and soon it helps you to build better circulation, health and increases your oxygen intake. A sound heart, like a sound car, can be driven far and fast without harm, but periods of rest and recovery are required. As we live longer, the need for rest generally increases, but not as much as most people imagine. A daily 30 minute nap is an ideal recharger after lunch.

Exercise Gives Huge Benefits for the Prevention of Heart Disease and also:

1. Tones muscles
2. Improves circulation
3. Lowers cholesterol
4. Chases depression
5. Eases stress
6. Stimulates internal organs
7. Improves sex
8. Promotes sound sleep
9. Helps you think better
10. Promotes deep breathing

Now Get Started – For Life is Precious

Start this very minute on your Heart Fitness Program! Get it firmly in your mind that you're going to build a fit heart! Banish all negative thoughts! Have faith . . . for you are now going to work with a powerful force – Mother Nature and God. Say to yourself day after day, I am building a healthy, strong, fit heart. Think strength and vitality for your heart. Take command of your body and mind today and let nothing distract you from following your Heart Fitness Program!

If you feel yourself weakening in your resolve, look to a Higher Power for courage and willpower. You were given one heart, one body, one life by your Creator . . . and you were given Mother Nature as your ally to help you achieve a long, healthy and happy life. But no one – not even God or Mother Nature – can make you help yourself, you must do it – so now get started!

The great thing in life is not so much where you stand, but in what direction you are moving – right (positive) or wrong (negative).

Chapter 10

Exercises For Heart Health and Good Circulation

Good Circulation – Key to Strong Heart

When any part of the circulatory system is seriously impaired, the billions of body cells it serves are deprived of their oxygen and nourishment. With their blood supply cut off, these cells will automatically break down. The cell damage may occur in the heart itself and in the brain, the lungs, kidneys, skin or other parts of the body. Remember – if you don't use your body, you will lose it!

Five Exercises for Increased Circulation

Exercise 1 – Windmill Exercise For Energy

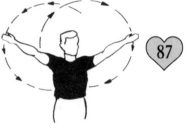

(A) Stand erect with heels and toes together, chest up, stomach drawn in, shoulders back, head high, with hands hanging loosely at your sides. Now, start swinging your arms in a forward circular motion then coming down along the sides of your body, continuing circles. Increase speed until you are making circles as fast as possible. Start by doing 10 circles forward and increase by several a day until you can bring it up to 30 circles at one time.

(B) Same position as above, only instead of making circles with the arms forward, make circles backward – in the opposite direction. Start with 10 and increase to 30.

Exercise 2 – Hands and Finger Circulation Exercise

Stand erect as in Exercise #1. Bring hands 10 inches in front of body at chest height, and from the wrists shake the relaxed hands vigorously. Do 15 shakes with both hands at the same time and then grip hands together 15 times. Now 15 times grip each hand individually into a tight fist, then relax the hands, stretching fingers out as far as possible.

Each day is God's gift to you. Make it blossom and grow into a thing of beauty.

Exercise 3 – Body Circulation-Builder

This exercise is great for people in cold climates to bring circulation to their arms, hands and upper body. Start in the same position as Exercise #1. Hold arms and hands outstretched horizontally at shoulder height. Each hand forms a half circle as the exercise is done. The right hand strikes the left shoulder and the left hand strikes the right shoulder at the same time. The arms are crisscrossed alternately with each repetition . . . right over left and then left over right. Slap the shoulders vigorously. Make it vigorous so each time the arms are flung open back to the starting position, then the chest is pushed forward and up. Start this exercise by doing it 10 times and work up until you can do it 30 times.

Exercise 4 – Leg and Feet Vibrating Exercise

Stand erect, feet about 8 to 10 inches apart and arms at sides. Now, put all your weight on your left foot and raise your right foot off the ground about 6 or 8 inches. Make short stretching kicks in a forward direction. (You may hold on to a chair.) You will feel vibration from the hips to the toes. Now alternate, standing on right foot and kicking with your left foot. Start with 10 kicks on each foot and increase the amount every day until you can kick about 30 times or more with each foot. Make this a vigorous exercise – it promotes great circulation to hips, thighs, calves and feet and is important for health.

Exercise 5 –Exercise for Blood Circulation in Head

Stand erect with knees relaxed and feet 12 inches apart. Lean forward from waist, with arms hanging down, relaxed near floor. (Hold on to chair if necessary.) In this position gently roll your head side to side and down and up. Do this exercise only a few times in beginning, until your neck and head becomes accustomed to more circulation.

These simple exercises cause no heart strain and are ideal for improving circulation. They help open up blocked arteries and blood vessels. When circulation is increased through exercise it helps purify the blood so more vital oxygen is carried to all parts of the body.

Exercise to Benefit the Liver and Kidneys

Your great filters – the kidneys – are the body's hardest working organs! Exercises that bend and twist the body at its middle will help to stimulate the kidneys, which makes them function more efficiently.

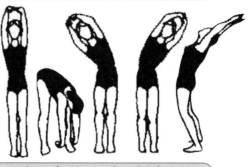

Here's a great exercise for stimulating the kidneys:

Stand up straight with hands over head. Now bend forward from waist with knees relaxed and try to touch toes. Return your hands overhead, now bend backwards as far as comfortable. Now, arms up, hands clasped, bend first to left side, then to right side as far as possible. Since most of the body's liquid waste is eliminated through the kidneys, you should do these kidney stimulating exercises daily. Start with 10 of each and work up to 30.

Exercises – Good For Heart, Nerves & Health   89

A normal, healthy heart cannot be injured by these exercises. Weak people should start slowly and work up to a vigorous workout. Just as exercise is good for any muscle, these circulatory exercises are beneficial for both a healthy and an injured heart. These exercises will condition your heart just as they do your visible muscles. Refuse to listen to people who try to frighten you away from exercise! The heart is a muscle and must be exercised if it is to remain strong. By exercising you will build a stronger heart and body!

Do these exercises daily – requires only 15 minutes. This is just a little time to invest in a healthy heart and a healthful life! If you have a sedentary job, if you spend a lot of time sitting or standing, do these exercises 2 or 3 times daily. When on long automobile drives, stop and do exercises every few hours. The more you do these exercises, the better circulation you will have, and this helps promote a stronger heart!

Nervous Tension can ruin your health in dozens of ways, diminish your productivity and even shorten your lifespan. – Dr. E. Jacobson, You Must Relax

The Dangers of Sitting too Long

Although most waste products are eliminated through the kidneys and colon, the lungs expel carbon dioxide. In the lungs tiny alveoli, blood discharges carbon dioxide and takes on oxygen, again turning a bright red. It then flows back into the heart, to be pumped out through the arteries to the rest of the body. This powerful cycle is repeated thousands of times daily. This is why you must never sit too long at one time. *Sitting slows down the circulation and stagnates the blood.* Long periods of sitting can be damaging to the heart. And please, never cross your legs – it's unhealthy!

People who sit too long may develop a thrombosis (blood clot) in the deep veins of the calf. If your office work requires sitting a lot, *get up and move around every hour.* On long car trips, stop every hour or so and take a walk or do some exercises. Remember when exercising, you flush out toxins and stimulate blood circulation through your vital pipes that supply food and oxygen.

The Art of Healthy Sitting

When sitting, please sit correctly! *The most disastrous and injurious habit of bad sitting is crossing the legs* for it compresses the popliteal artery in back of knees which can cause a variety of unhealthy problems (blood stagnation in hip, leg, knee, feet and backaches, varicose veins, hemorrhoids, headaches, pain, etc.).

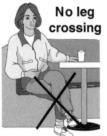
No leg crossing

When you sit in a chair, sit well back. Do not let the edge of the chair cut off circulation in the back of the knees. Keep your feet on floor. Dangling your legs puts too much pressure on veins. When I was small, my dad shortened the legs of a table for me so that my feet would touch the floor. Adults who have shorter legs should use a box or footstool. We love rocking chairs – you can get rest by sitting, plus peaceful (problem solving) rocking exercise!

A strong body makes a strong mind. – Thomas Jefferson, 3rd U.S. President, 1801-1809

When we lose one blessing, another is unexpectedly given in its place. – C.S. Lewis

Exercise (Sweating) is Healthy for You!

The skin, with its millions of pores and sweat glands, is the body's largest eliminating organ – (often called the third kidney). Sweat has a dual purpose – it rids the body of impurities and serves as a temperature regulator. When our body is exposed to heat or *warmed up* by exercise, sweat glands are stimulated into action. Evaporation of the sweat cools the blood when it reaches the skin. This helps the body from becoming overheated and, at the same time, eliminates impurities near the skin's surface.

It's the toxic impurities or the mixture with skin dirt, that gives sweat a bad odor. If you are clean inside and out, then there is only the good sweat smell. Regardless of what deodorant advertisers say, *it's healthy to sweat*. From dancing, calisthenics, walking, cycling and even vigorous housework, to saunas and steam rooms – any activity that makes you sweat improves your heart action and health. Hard work never hurts when you're healthy!

Indulge in Hobbies that are Active and Fun

My dad said if he were the President of the United States he would advocate laws requiring all people who work sitting down to spend an equal amount of time in keeping physically fit by brisk walking, etc. Also TV or computer addicts would be required to spend an hour in brisk walking for every hour they sit before a screen.

We would like to start a healthy-heart crusade against inactivity, long sitting and sedentary activities. Long sitting slows down circulation and when that happens many changes take place in the artery walls. You must keep active! When you relax, relax actively. Cultivate hobbies that give you needed exercise that you can enjoy such as hiking, swimming, tennis, golf, etc. You can't build a strong heart unless you exercise, walk briskly, bend, twist, vibrate your body, which promotes healthy overall body circulation. Remember stagnation breeds disease.

To maintain good health the body must be exercised properly (walking, jogging, running, biking, swimming, deep breathing, good posture, etc.) and nourished wisely (healthy foods), so as to provide and increase the good life of radiant health, joy, peace and happiness. – Paul C. Bragg, ND, PhD.

Avoid Constricting Clothes and Shoes

Anything that impedes blood circulation damages the heart and its arterial and vascular systems. Therefore, wear no constricting undergarments – this includes tight bras,* belts, collars, ties and above all, tight shoes.

Tight shoes can do more to disturb the circulation than any other article of clothing because the feet must always be well supplied with blood. There are 26 bones in each foot – more than in any other part of the body. When the blood does not reach the feet in the required quantities, toxins are retained in the cell structures of the feet. That is why so many people's feet have an unpleasant odor – they need to detoxify their body.

Many unhealthy conditions of stiffness, deformities and pain are brought on by ill-fitting shoes that cause poor circulation and incorrect posture when walking and standing! Only wear comfortable, practical shoes that don't bind or inhibit the free blood circulation in the feet.

Exercise Helps Build Better Circulation To Your Feet, Hands and Whole Body

Walking barefoot is the ideal way to walk. Each time we remove our shoes and walk barefoot is an opportunity to improve our circulation and walk toward more fitness for our heart. Walking or light jogging on grass, sand, the earth or simply walking barefoot around the house improves circulation with each step and helps strengthen the heart!

The heart must pump blood to the legs and feet, as well as to the arms and hands. Most people do not have sufficient rhythmic circulation to these extremities. That is why so many people complain of cold feet and legs that *go to sleep* easily and arms and hands that become cold and numb. Following is a hydro-therapeutic water therapy that helps alleviate these conditions.

*Read "Dressed to Kill", by Sydney Singer, on breast cancer and bra studies. Available from: www.Amazon.com
(My father insisted – I've never worn a bra, only a chemise. – Patricia Bragg)

Slow down and enjoy life. It's not only the scenery you miss by going too fast – you also miss the sense of where you're going and why! – Eddie Cantor

Cold and Hot Water Circulation Therapy:

Get 2 foot tubs or wash tubs. Fill one with hot water – about 104° or as hot as you can stand. Fill the other with cold water, preferably with ice cubes added. Now for 2 minutes put your feet in the hot water and your entire lower arms (hands to elbows) submerged in the cold water. After 2 minutes reverse the procedure – put your feet in the cold water, your arms and hands in the hot water for another 2 minute period. Repeat this cycle 5 times, then take a coarse cotton towel and rub your feet, arms and hands vigorously until they are warm and glowing with tingling, healthy circulation.

Here's another super therapy to stimulate circulation in the feet. Sit on a chair next to a bathtub with feet dangling over the tub; turn on a strong flow of water and for 5 minutes, alternate hot and cold water over your feet. Finish up with a coarse towel rub and massage.

Special Shower Builds Healthy Circulation

Here's a progressive method for improving circulation over your entire body. All you need is a large back brush or Swedish bath friction mitt, castile soap and a coarse Turkish towel. Get into shower and turn on the hot water. With brush or mitt, gently scrub your body. At first your coddled body won't be able to take too much scrubbing. Also it's good to hand–massage your body, neck and shoulders. After your scrub/massage part, alternate hot and cold showers every 2 to 3 minutes.* Now towel rub dry your body for 3 to 5 minutes – your circulation will tingle!

It's wonderful relaxation for tired or sore muscles and refreshing stimulation with the hot/cold water shower, letting the spray beat heavily on back and shoulders. Occasionally before shower apply Bragg Olive Oil if skin is dry. We advise this relaxing shower before dinner on days when you come home tired. It refreshes and relaxes you.

---

*Use a filtered shower head to remove chlorine, lead, mercury, arsenic, iron, hydrogen sulfide, bacteria, fungi, dirt and sediment from your water. To get best shower filter call weekdays 800-446-1990. I have been using this shower filter for 5 years and enjoy my chlorine-free showers! – Patricia Bragg, ND, PhD.

Great Framingham 50 Year Heart Study

In 1948 in Framingham, Massachusetts, 2,336 men and 2,873 women participated in a landmark study, the Framingham Heart Study. This ongoing study is still the source of much of our present understanding of heart disease and stroke. The original study group of 1948 and the succeeding generation of Framingham residents have been followed throughout their lives. Everyone has been interviewed every 2 years for over 50 years. This massive pioneer medical research continues today.

In 1971, the original Framingham subjects were joined by 5,135 of their children. The researchers were pleased to find a 43% reduction in heart disease deaths from the 1948 group. *The New England Journal of Medicine* says the increasing heart-health of Framingham's 1970's test group is primarily the result of the lifestyle improvements (reducing cholesterol, blood pressure and stop smoking factors) that so harmed the early 1950's group. See web: *framingham.com/heart.*

Dr. T. Colin Campbell's China Project

94

In another landmark study, the China Project, written by Dr. T. Colin Campbell, the effects of nearly 50 disease categories on counties in US and China were observed for 20 years. Results showed that populations using a diet richer in animal products and higher in total fat were much more afflicted with chronic degenerative diseases (cancers, cardiovascular diseases, diabetes, etc.). The Chinese diet contains 0 to 20% animal-based foods, while the affluent American diet, *sad to say*, is comprised of 50 to 70%. What's worse, far more Americans are clinically obese, even though the Chinese consume 30% more total calories! Another astonishing fact is that China's high cholesterol levels are almost equal to the U.S.'s low! For more info on this study, see web: *www.nutrition.cornell.edu/ChinaProject.com.*

What these 2 ambitious studies have to say about maintaining cardiovascular health is just what we've been telling people for years! Eat a natural diet low in fats, cholesterol, sugars, salts, etc.; exercise regularly; fast; don't smoke – this is The Bragg Healthy Lifestyle!

I live on legumes, vegetables & fruits. No dairy, no meat of any kind, no chicken, no turkey, & very little fish, once in a while. It changed my metabolism & I lost 24 pounds. I did research & found 82% of people who go on a plant-based diet begin to heal themselves, as I did. – U.S. President Bill Clinton, 1993-2001

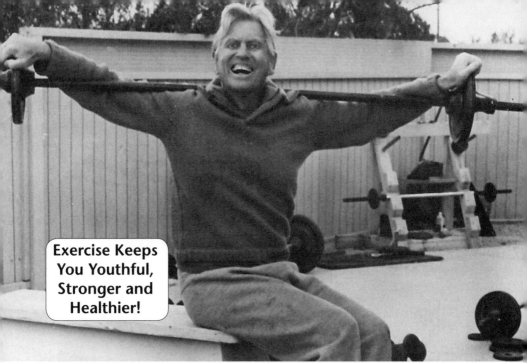

> **Exercise Keeps You Youthful, Stronger and Healthier!**

Paul C. Bragg and Patricia lift weights 3 times weekly.

Iron-Pumping Oldsters (ages 86 to 96) Triple Their Muscle Strength In Landmark U.S. Government Study

WASHINGTON, June 13, 1990 – Ageing nursing home residents in Boston *pumping iron?* Elderly weightlifters tripling and quadrupling their muscle strength? Is it possible? Most people would doubt and wonder at this amazing revelation!

Yet government experts on ageing answered those questions with a resounding *yes* according to results of a new study. They turned a group of frail Boston nursing home residents, aged 86 to 96, into weightlifters to demonstrate that it's never too late to reverse age-related declines in muscle strength. The study group participated in a regime of high-intensity weight-training in research conducted by the Agriculture Departments Human Research Center of Ageing at Tufts University in Boston. *A high-intensity weight training program is capable of inducing dramatic increases in muscle strength in frail men and women up to 96 years of age,* reported by the study director, Dr. Maria A. Fiatarone.

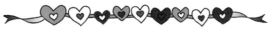

There is no thrill quite like doing something you didn't know you could.
– Marjorie Holmes (find her books on Amazon.com)

Despite their many handicaps, the elderly weightlifters increased their muscle strength by 3-4 times as much in as little as 8 weeks. Fiatarone said they probably were stronger at the end of the program than they had been in years! See web: *www.framinghamheartstudy.org.*

Fiatarone and her associates emphasized the safety of such a closely supervised weight lifting program, even among people in frail health. The average age of the 10 participants was 90. Six had coronary heart disease, 7 had arthritis, 6 had bone fractures resulting from osteoporosis, 4 had high blood pressure, and all had been physically inactive for years. Yet no serious medical problems resulted from this program. A few of the participants did report minor muscle and joint aches, but 9 of the 10 still completed the program. One man, aged 86, felt a pulling sensation at the site of a previous hernia incision and dropped out after 4 weeks.

The study participants, drawn from a 712 bed long-term care facility in Boston, worked out 3 times a week during the study. They performed 3 sets of 8 repetitions with each leg on a weight lifting machine. The weights were gradually increased from 10 lbs. to 40 lbs. at the end of the 8 week program. (*jcaaa.org/liftingweights.htm*)

Muscle strength in the average adult decreases by 30% - 50% during the course of a lifetime. Muscle atrophy and weakness is not merely a cosmetic problem in elderly people, but especially the frail elderly. Researchers have linked muscle weakness with recurrent falls, which is a major cause of immobility and death with the American elderly. This is costing the U.S. billions of dollars yearly in staggering medical fees.

Previous studies have suggested that weight training can be helpful in reversing age-related muscle weakness. But Fiatarone said physicians have been reluctant to recommend weight lifting for frail elderly patients with multiple health problems. This 1990 government study should help to change their minds. This shows the importance of keeping the 640 body muscles as active and fit as possible to maintain general good physical fitness and good heart and body health.

When you increase strength training, brisk walking becomes easier. That lets you walk faster and farther, which gives the heart and lungs a better workout.

Chapter 11

Doctor Pure Water

Pure Water Helps Keep Body Clean Inside

To have a clean, healthy bloodstream and arteries free of corrosion, we must not only eat correctly but also drink the right fluids. *The liquids which go into our bodies must be pure and nourishing.* To begin with, we believe that every person should have the equivalent of *8-10 glasses purified or distilled water every day.* It can be obtained in most supermarkets, grocery stores and health stores. If you cannot find it readily, look under *water* in the yellow pages of your telephone directory for local bottled water suppliers.

Distilled water has no inorganic minerals to deposit on the walls of the arteries and other *pipes* of the body. In contrast, most sources of *well, spring and river waters all contain inorganic minerals and some even have toxic chemicals which cannot ever be utilized in the body chemistry.* They can corrode the human *pipes* just as they do the plumbing pipes which bring water into your home.

97

Hard Water Causes Hard Arteries

The human body has a vast piping system called the bloodstream. A healthy heart must have clean, open coronary arteries. The blood must be able to flow through them smoothly to nourish the heart and keep it pumping steadily and efficiently (it is our miracle muscle pump).

Suppose a person drinks only the hard chemicalized water (as most people do) and their pipelines become clogged and blocked by the inorganic minerals which can not be absorbed into the body. Blockage in the coronary arteries feeding the heart, reduces the amount of blood reaching the heart. When the blood supply is reduced enough, the affected parts of the heart cease to function. A heart attack and even death may result when some sections of the heart muscle stop functioning.

Drinking water at correct times maximizes effectiveness on Body:

2 glasses purified/distilled water in morning helps activate internal organs.
Glass water with vinegar 30 minutes before meals, helps digestion & Gerds.
Glass of water before taking a bath or shower helps lower blood pressure.
Glass of water 2 hours before bedtime helps avoid stroke & heart attack.

The Difference Between Organic and Inorganic Minerals

Inorganic minerals never lived and are inert . . . which means that they *cannot be absorbed into the body!*

Organic minerals are those which come from that which is *living* or has lived . . . and *16 of these organic minerals are essential elements of the human body.* When we eat an apple or any other fruit or vegetable, that substance is living, for it has a certain lifespan after it has been picked. The same is true of animal foods, such as fish, milk, cheese and eggs. Animals obtain their organic minerals from plants. We humans obtain our organic minerals from both plants and animals.

Only a living plant has the power to extract inorganic minerals from the earth and sun and change them into organic minerals. No animal or human can do this. If you were stranded on an uninhabited island where nothing was growing, you would starve to death. Although the soil beneath your feet would contain all 16 *essential* minerals, your body could not absorb them.

Organic minerals are vital in keeping us alive and healthy, but inorganic minerals can stiffen, sicken and can slowly kill us!

Many years ago my father was on an expedition in China when one part of the country was suffering from drought and famine. He saw the poor, starving people heating and eating dirt for want of food. They died horrible deaths because they could not get one bit of nourishment from the inorganic minerals of the earth.

WATER IS KEY TO HEALTH & ALL BODY FUNCTIONS:

- Heart
- Circulation
- Digestion
- Bones & Joints
- Muscles
- Metabolism
- Assimilation
- Elimination
- Nerves
- Energy
- Sex
- Glands

Pure water is the best drink for a wise man. – Henry David Thoreau

Distilled water plays vital part in treatment of illness, arthritis, etc. – Dr. Banik

Most Americans' bodies thirst for pure distilled water! Their bodies become sick, prematurely aged, crippled and stiff due to inorganic minerals and chemicalized water and lack of sufficient pure water!

Hard Water is Unhealthy

For years we've heard people claim that certain waters were rich in all the minerals. What minerals are they talking about? Inorganic or organic? If they are inorganic, people are simply burdening their bodies with inert minerals which may cause the development of stones in the kidneys and gallbladder and acid crystals in the arteries, veins, joints and other parts of the body.

Dad was reared in a part of Virginia known for its extremely *hard water*. The drinking water was heavily saturated with inorganic minerals – especially sodium, iron and calcium. He saw many of his adult relations and friends die of kidney trouble. Nearly all the people were prematurely old because the inorganic minerals had collected on the inner walls of their arteries and veins. These people would often die from hardening of the arteries. One of Dad's uncles died at the great Johns Hopkins Hospital in Baltimore, Maryland, when he was only 48 years of age. The doctors who performed the autopsy stated that his arteries were so corroded with inorganic minerals that they were as hard as clay pipes!

Vegetable and Fruit Juices Contain Mother Nature's Distilled Water

No new water has been put on the face of Mother Earth since it was originally formed. Just as the same energy is formed and re-formed, so the same water is used and re-used over and over again by the miracle of Mother Nature. Waters of the earth are purified by distillation. The sun evaporates the water which is collected into clouds. When the clouds become full we have rain and dew – pure, perfectly clean, distilled water, free of all harmful inorganic substances, until polluted!

Years ago when late actor Douglas Fairbanks, Senior, and Dad were close friends, they roamed the South Sea Islands for several months. During that trip Dad came upon an island inhabited by *beautiful, healthy Polynesians* who drank only distilled water because the island was surrounded by the Pacific Ocean. Their island was based on porous coral which could not hold water – so they would *only drink rain water* or the fresh, clear, clean water of the green coconut. Dad had never seen any finer specimens of humanity than these native South Sea Islanders. There were several doctors on the yacht who thoroughly examined the most mature people on these islands. One heart doctor stated that he had never in his life examined such healthy, well-preserved people.

You may have noted we said only the most mature people were examined by the doctors. *They were so completely unaware of age* that no such word existed in their language! They never celebrated birthdays, so they were forever young – gloriously ageless, not only in years but in body. These older men performed as well in the vigorous native dances as the younger men. They were all beautiful human specimens because they lived their lengthy lives drinking only pure distilled water, eating natural foods and enjoying a healthy lifestyle.

Why We Drink Only Distilled Water

100

Sadly, in some areas it's no longer safe to drink rain or snow water because of man's vast reach of polluting the air. But when you drink the fresh juices of fruits and vegetables, remember that all of this liquid has been *distilled by Mother Nature* and is 100% inorganic mineral-free. Fresh fruit and vegetable juices contain Mother Nature's pure distilled water, plus important nutrients such as natural sugars, organic minerals and vitamins.

You will hear people say, *distilled water is dead water, a fish cannot live in it.* Of course a fish cannot live in distilled water for any length of time! It needs the vegetation that grows in rivers, lakes and seas. But this doesn't mean it isn't the very best of all waters for humans to drink.

Another erroneous distilled water notion is that it *leaches the organic minerals out of the body.* This is 100% false! It leaches out inorganic minerals which you want to be rid of that can cause you painful health problems.

It's excellent for detoxification – distilled water helps to dissolve and flush out the terrible toxic poisons that collect in the bodies of modern man. This pure water helps to eliminate these toxic poisons through the kidneys without creating painful problems that inorganic pebbles and stones do!

Every liquid prescription that is mixed in any drug store the world over is prepared with distilled water. It is used in baby formulas and for many hundreds of other purposes where absolutely pure water is essential.

Distilled water is soft water. If you wash your hair in distilled water you will discover how soft it is. Water softeners are being used in millions of homes because hard water is not ideal for washing clothes, dishes, etc. Please do not drink the water out of water softeners! It's not healthy for drinking or cooking because of its salt and chemical content.

At the Bragg home we have a water distiller and for our office staff we have distilled water delivered in 5 gallon bottles. Try distilled water exclusively for a year, you will see the results and never want to drink hard water again!

The body is 70% water and pure, steam-distilled (chemical-free) water is important for total health. You should drink at least 8 glasses of water daily. Read our book, *Water – The Shocking Truth*, for more info on the importance of pure water. See back pages for book list.

Pure, distilled water is vitally important in following The Bragg Healthy Lifestyle. Water is the key to all body functions including: digestion, circulation, bones and joints, assimilation, elimination, muscles, nerves, glands, sex and senses. The right kind of water is one of your best natural protections against all kinds of diseases and viral infections, such as influenza and pneumonia. It is a vital factor in all body fluids, tissues, cells, lymph, blood and all glandular secretions. Water holds all nutritive factors in solution, as well as toxins and body wastes, and acts as the main transportation medium throughout the body, for both nutritional and cleansing purposes!

Distilled water is the world's purest and best water!

Water from chemically treated public water systems – and even from many wells and springs – is likely to be loaded with poisonous chemicals and toxic trace elements. Depending upon the kinds of pipes used in the buildings, the water is likely to be overloaded with lead (from older, soldered pipe joints), zinc (from old-fashioned galvanized pipes) or with copper and cadmium (from copper pipes). These trace elements are released in dangerous quantities by the chemical action of the water flowing against the metals of the pipes.

The 70% Watery Human

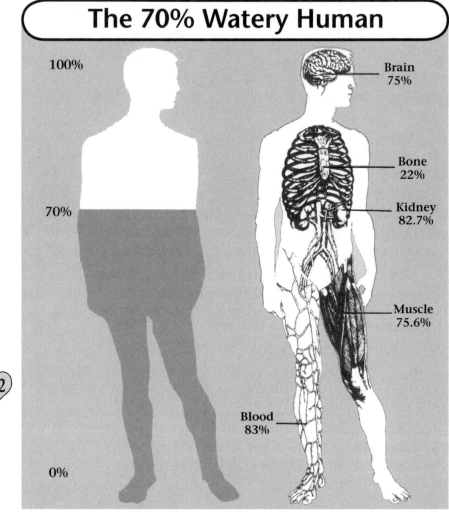

100%

Brain
75%

Bone
22%

Kidney
82.7%

70%

Muscle
75.6%

102

Blood
83%

0%

The amount of water in the human body, averaging 70%, varies considerably and even from one part of the body to another area (illustration on right). A lean man may hold 70% of his weight in body water, while a woman – because of her larger proportion of water-poor fatty tissues – may be only 52% water. The lowering of the water content in the blood is what triggers the hypothalamus, the brain's vital thirst center, to send out its familiar urgent demand for a drink of water! Please obey and drink ample amounts (8 glasses) of purified water daily. *By the time you feel thirsty, you're already dehydrated. – American Running & Fitness Association*

Water Percentage in Various Body Parts:

Teeth	10%	Lungs	80%
Bones	22%	Brain	75%
Cartilage	55%	Bile	86%
Red blood corpuscles	68.7%	Plasma	90%
Liver	71.5%	Blood	83%
Muscle tissue	75%	Lymph	94%
Spleen	75.5%	Saliva	95.5%

This chart shows why 8-10 glasses of water daily is important.

Ten Common Sense Reasons Why You Should Only Drink Pure, Distilled Water!

- There are over 12,000 toxic chemicals on the market today . . . and 500 are being added yearly! Wherever you live, in the city or on the farm, some of these chemicals are getting into your drinking water. Beware of chemicalized water.

- No one on the face of the earth today knows what effect these chemicals have on the body as they blend into thousands of different combinations. It is like making a mixture of colors; one drop could change the color.

- Proper equipment hasn't been designed yet to detect some of these chemicals, and may not be for years to come.

- The miracle working body is made up of 70% water. Therefore, don't you think you should be particular, wise and cautious about the type of water you drink?

- The Navy has been drinking distilled water for years!

- Distilled water is chemical and mineral free. Distillation removes all the chemicals and impurities from water that are possible to remove. If distillation doesn't remove them, there is no known method today that will.

- The body does need minerals . . . but it is not necessary that they come from water. There is not one mineral in water which cannot be found more abundantly in food! Water is the most unreliable source of minerals because it varies from one area to another. The food we eat – not the water we drink – is the best source of organic minerals!

- Distilled water is used for intravenous feeding, inhalation therapy, prescriptions and baby formulas. Therefore, doesn't it make sense that it is good for everyone?

- Thousands of water distillers have been sold throughout the United States and around the world to individuals, families, dentists, doctors, hospitals, nursing homes and government agencies. These informed, alert consumers are helping protect their health by using only steam distilled water. They don't want the toxic, harmful chemicals.

- With chemicals, pollutants and other impurities in our water, it makes good sense to clean up the water you drink using Mother Nature's inexpensive way – distillation.

Pure distilled water is truly god's greatest gift to us – it's the vital natural chemistry of life, and a source of health. – Paul C. Bragg

Fluorine is a Deadly Poison!

Millions of innocent people have been brainwashed by the aluminum companies to erroneously believe that adding sodium fluoride (their waste by-product) to our drinking water will reduce tooth decay in our children. Americans get sodium fluoride in their drinking water without thinking about it. Sodium fluorine, a chemical "cousin" of sodium fluoride, is used as a rat and roach killer and a deadly pesticide. Yet this deadly sodium fluoride, injected almost by government edict into drinking water in the proportion of 1.2 parts per million (PPM), has been declared by the US Public Health Service to be *safe for all human consumption.* Every chemist knows that such *absolute safety* is not only false and is truly unattainable, but a total illusion!

Keep Toxic Fluoride Out of Your Water!

Most of the water Americans drink has fluoride in it, including tap, bottled and canned drinks and foods! The ADA (American Dental Association) is insisting that the FDA (Food and Drug Association) mandate the addition of toxic fluoride to all bottled waters! Defend your right to drink pure, non-fluoridated tap and bottled waters! Challenge and stop local and state water fluoridation policies! Call, write, fax or e-mail all your state officials and Congress people and send them a copy of this book.

104

CHECK FOLLOWING WEBSITES FOR FLUORIDE UPDATES:

- www.voteoutfluoride.com
- www.FluorideAlert.org
- www.FluorideResearch.org
- www.Bruha.com/fluoride
- www.bragg.com
- www.fluoridation.com
- www.Keepers-of-the-Well.org
- www.dentalwellness4u.com/oralhealth/fluoride.html

These Eleven Major American Associations
Stopped Endorsing Water Fluoridation back in 1996

- *American Heart Association*
- *American Cancer Society*
- *American Diabetes Association*
- *American Civil Liberties Union*
- *American Chiropractic Association*
- *Society of Toxicology*
- *National Kidney Foundation*
- *American Psychiatric Association*
- *American Academy of Allergy & Immunology*
- *Chronic Fatigue Syndrome Action Network*
- *Nat'l Institute of Law Municipal Officers*

Showers, Toxic Chemicals & Chlorine

Water chlorination has been widely used to "purify" water in this country for most of this century. But its negative effects on health surely outweigh any benefits. "Chlorine is the greatest crippler and killer of modern times. While it prevented epidemics of one disease, it was creating another. Twenty years after the start of chlorinating our drinking water in 1904, the present mounting epidemic of heart trouble, cancer and senility began and is costing billions."
– Dr. Joseph Price, *Coronaries/Cholesterol/Chlorine*

Skin absorption of toxic dangerous contaminants has been greatly underestimated and the ingestion may not constitute the sole primary route of exposure.
– Dr. Halina Brown, *American Journal of Public Health*

Taking long hot showers is a health risk, according to the latest research. Showers – and to a lesser extent baths – lead to a greater exposure to toxic chemicals contained in water supplies than does drinking the water. These toxic chemicals evaporate out of the water and are inhaled. They can also spread through the house and be inhaled by others. People get six to 100 times more chemicals by breathing the air while taking showers and baths than they would by drinking the water. – Ian Anderson, *New Scientist*

A Professor of Water Chemistry at the University of Pittsburgh claims that exposure to vaporized chemicals in the water through showering, bathing and inhalation is 100 times greater than through drinking the chemicals in water.
– *The Nader Report – Troubled Waters on Tap*

Angina, allergies, asthma, back and joint pains, migraines, stomach pains and arthritis may be symptoms of severe dehydration – which is easily helped by drinking 8 to 10 glasses of purified distilled water daily! Start increasing your water intake today. Be water wise and health safe! – Paul C. Bragg

There is only one water that is clean & that is steam distilled water. No other substance on our planet does so much to keep us healthy & get us well as distilled water does. – Dr. James Balch, Co-Author, *Dietary Wellness* (amazon.com)

Don't gamble with your health, use a shower filter to remove toxins. Info on best shower filter available, call weekdays, 800-446-1990. I have been using this filter for 5 years and enjoy my safe, chlorine-free showers! - PB

Five Hidden Toxic Dangers in Your Shower:

● **Chlorine:** Added to all municipal water supplies, this disinfectant hardens arteries, destroys proteins in the body, irritates skin and sinus conditions and aggravates any asthma, allergies and respiratory problems.

● **Chloroform:** This powerful by-product of chlorination causes excessive free radical formation (a cause of accelerated ageing! see page 25-26), normal cells to mutate and cholesterol to form. It's a known carcinogen!

● **DCA (Dichloroacedic acid):** This chlorine by-product alters cholesterol metabolism and has been shown to cause liver cancer in lab animals.

● **MX (toxic chlorinated acid):** Another by-product of chlorination, MX is known to cause genetic mutations that can lead to cancer growth and has been found in all chlorinated water for which it was tested.

● **Proven cause of bladder and rectal cancer:** Research proved that chlorinated water is the direct cause of 9% of all U.S. bladder cancers and 15% of all rectal cancers.

106

Don't Gamble With Your Health – Use Shower Filter That Removes Toxins

The most effective method of removing hazards from your shower is the quick and easy installation of a filter on your shower arm. The best filter we found removes chlorine, lead, mercury, iron, chlorine by-products, arsenic, hydrogen sulfide, and many other unseen toxic contaminants, such as bacteria, fungi, dirt and sediments. It has a 12 to 18 month filter life-span and the filter is easily cleaned by backwashing and replaced when needed. I have been using this filter for 5 years and really enjoy my chlorine-free showers! For more info on buying the best shower filter call (800) 446-1990 weekdays.

Start enjoying safe, chlorine-free showers right away. It's essential to reducing your risk of heart disease and cancer and to ease the strain on your immune system. And you may even get rid of long-standing conditions – from sinus and respiratory problems to dry, itchy skin.

Kind words are the music of the world . . . as if they were some angel's song which has lost its way and come to Earth. – Fredrick William Faber

You Get More Toxic Exposure from Taking a Chlorinated Water Shower Than From Drinking the Same Water!

Two of the very highly toxic and volatile chemicals, trichloroethylene and chloroform, have been proven as toxic contaminants found in most all municipal drinking water supplies. The National Academy of Sciences recently has estimated that hundreds of people die in the United States each year from the cancers caused largely by ingesting water pollutants from inhalation as air pollutants in the home. Inhalation exposure to water pollutants is largely ignored. Recent shocking data indicates that hot showers can liberate about 50% of the chloroform and 80% of the trichloroethylene into the air.

Tests show your body can absorb more toxic chlorine from a 10 minute shower than drinking 8 glasses of the same water. How can that be? A warm shower opens up your pores, causing your skin to act like a sponge. As a result, you not only inhale the toxic chlorine vapors, you absorb them through your skin, directly into your bloodstream – at a toxic rate that is up to 6 times higher than drinking it.

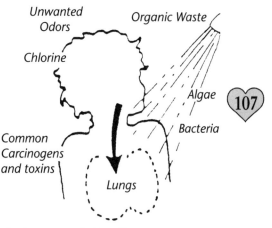

In terms of cumulative damage to your health, showering in chlorinated water is one of the most dangerous risks you take daily. Short-term risks include: eyes, sinus, throat, skin and lung irritation. Long-term risks include: excessive free radical formation (that ages you!), higher vulnerability to genetic mutation and cancer development; and difficulty metabolizing cholesterol that can cause hardened arteries. – Science News

The treatment of diseases should go to the root of the cause. Often it is found in severe dehydration from lack of purified water, and an unhealthy lifestyle!

Distillation effectively removes the widest variety of toxins and contaminants from water. David & Anne Frahm, *Healthy Habits*

Comparison of Water Treatment Methods
Steam Distilled Water is the Best!

POLLUTANT	Filter Sediment	Filter Carbon	Deionization	Reverse Osmosis	Steam Distillation
Arsenic	○	○	●	●	●
Bacteria	○	○	○	◑	●
Cadmium	○	○	●	●	●
Calcium	○	○	●	●	●
Chlorides	○	○	●	●	●
Chlorine	○	●	○	●[1]	●[1]
Cryptosporidium	○	○	○	●	●
Detergents	○	◑	●	●	●
Fluorides	○	○	●	●	●
Lead	○	○	●	●	●
Magnesium	○	○	●	●	●
Nitrate	○	○	◑	◑	●
Organics	○	●	○	●[1]	●[1]
Pesticides	○	●	○	●[1]	●[1]
Phosphates	○	○	●	●	●
Radon	○	○	●	●	●
Sediment	●	◑	●	●	●
Sodium	○	○	●	●	●
Sulfates	○	◑	●	●	●
Viruses	○	○	○	○	●

○ Ineffective or No Reduction   ◑ Significant Reduction   ● Complete or Significant Reduction

1 – A Carbon Filter Needed (The best home distillers have also carbon filters.)

For info on reasonable water distillers & shower head filters for your home that will remove harmful chemicals from your water call weekdays (800) 446-1990

Chapter 12

Doctor Healthy Foods

Importance of Balanced Body Chemistry

In this "Bragg Heart Fitness Program" we have been emphasizing the *dont's* because we consider these much more difficult to follow than the *do's*. Now we will detail what kind of food program you should follow for heart fitness, health and living a longer healthier life.

Every time you plan a meal, check off these items on the fingers of your hand to see if you are eating a *nutritionally well-balanced combination of foods: protein, carbohydrates, fats, fruits and vegetables.*

Protein: Building Blocks of the Body

Protein foods are raw nuts, seeds (such as sunflower, sesame, pumpkin), Bragg Nutritional Yeast Seasoning, wheat germ, soybeans, dairy products, whole grain cereals, meat, fish, poultry and protein supplements. Protein is one of the most important food elements and *is essential for keeping the heart fit.* You must have protein for building every cell of your body. This fundamental demand of Mother Nature rules every creature living on the face of the Earth, including man.

Protein is you – flesh, muscle, blood, heart, bones, skin and hair – all the components of the body are essentially composed of protein. *You are literally "built" of protein.* This basic function of your body – of converting food into living tissue – is one of life's miracles. Your life processes and the factors that help you resist disease are all composed of protein (amino acids) components.

Every time you move a muscle, every time your heart beats, every time you breathe, you consume protein in the form of amino acids. The link between protein and body tissue is the amino acids – and the bloodstream carries them to every part of the body where they work to repair, rebuild and maintain body tissues. They enrich blood and condition the organs, including the heart.

Poor diet & lack of exercise may soon be the leading causes of death in U.S.
See website: www.nutrition.gov for healthy nutritional tips

Amino Acids – The Body's Building Blocks

The body's human tissue is renewed daily. Scientists once believed that there were great masses of protein in the body in an inactive state – stores of protein built up in the muscles, tissues and organs which remain there until the body might need them. Now we know that the great builder protein is not stationary, but in motion. This activity requires a replenishment of essential protein for the rebuilding process, especially in older people.

What is connection between Amino Acids and proteins? Amino Acids are the important miracle building blocks from which different food proteins are constructed. When we eat a protein food, such as meat or soybeans, the natural hydrochloric acid in the stomach *digests* the protein, releasing the Aminos Acids. They are the link between the food we eat and assimilate for our body's tissues. Amino Acids are what makes our food turn into us!

Unlike vitamins, the *activators* in our nutrition, Amino Acids actually enter into the structure of the body tissue itself. They are the very foundation of all protein foods. They build muscles, tissues and organs and circulate freely in the blood – the body's vital lifestream. Your blood is your precious river of life – protect it!

The phytonutrients found in soy are specifically known as isoflavins. These isoflavins have been shown to be strong antioxidants that help repair cellular damage in the body, and they have anti-tumor effects. Soy can contribute to optimal health and has remarkable health-promoting properties. See phytochemical chart on page 118.

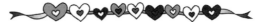

WHAT ARE AMINO ACIDS? *They're the building blocks of all our organs and tissues. They are the building blocks of proteins. They are essential for production of energy within ourselves, for detoxification and for the vital transmission of nerve impulses. In short, they are the very soup of life, and are almost always overlooked and neglected.* – H.J. Hoegerman, M.D., (Bragg Aminos Fan)

Amino Acids are needed for building every part of the body: bones, blood, hair, skin, nails and glands – and are Mother Nature's and God's life-giving secret to a long life. – Paul C. Bragg, ND, PhD., Originator of Health Stores

Each day, time is your greatest treasure, spend it wisely! – Patricia Bragg, ND, PhD.

Amino Acids – Life-Givers & Life-Extenders

Famous Pioneer Endocrinologist and Biochemist, Dr. W. Donner Denckla, with the National Institute of Health, has been immersed in pathfinding research on longevity for years. Dr. Denckla has the opinion that ageing is not inevitable and that Amino Acids and their interaction with a hormone secreted by the pituitary gland seem to be the key to slowing down ageing.

If we could look within the body, we would see all the living cells that make up the tissues, organs and bloodstream are in a highly active state. Paul C. Bragg was the first to preach the gospel of Amino Acids, their relationship to ageing and how they can help keep you younger, longer! He stressed that when the protein supply – the Amino Acids – are replenished regularly, the new cells that are constantly growing and being born can then thrive and live with more positive intensity! Another important benefit of Amino Acids – they help form antibodies to fight germs, infections and disease!

Bragg Introduces Miracles of Soybeans

Over 88 years ago my father introduced Bragg Liquid Aminos to the health-minded as a way to help them increase natural, life-building vegetable protein intake in a form that's easily digestible and delicious to use! It's a liquid form of soy protein from pure, healthy (certified non-genetically engineered) soybeans – a 100% health product that contains no coloring agents, preservatives or added sodium. Lack of adequate Amino Acids in your body may make it impossible for the vitamins and minerals to perform their specific duties. Amino Acids are inseparably interwoven with vitamins and minerals for good sound nutrition. Bragg Liquid Aminos contains no meat, and adds delicious natural flavors and zest to most all foods by sprinkling or spraying on foods. It's the most delicious, nutritious and unique gourmet health seasoning, for it contains 16 important vital Amino Acids and Isoflavins for super health.

Up to 90% of deaths annually are self-inflicted by an unhealthy lifestyle!

Let food be your medicine, and medicine be your food. – Hippocrates

The Importance of Soy Lecithin

The liver performs over five hundred separate jobs – one is producing the body's normal cholesterol and an important substance called lecithin. Lecithin is one of God's greatest gifts to man! It mixes with bile in the gallbladder and is emptied along with the bile into the small intestine to help in digestion of fats as they leave the stomach. Lecithin is a fat homogenizing agent which breaks up fat into tiny particles. One of the great health discoveries of Nutritional Science is the role of lecithin (from soybeans) in helping the body to dispose of these excessive fats! You can see that a deficiency of lecithin may cause serious coronary blockage problems. (We use lecithin granules like butter over veggies, potatoes, and add to our pep drinks, etc., see inside front cover.)

The soybean is the richest source of lecithin. It's also found in all products which contain fat, such as the germ (part that sprouts) of various grains. Lecithin and wheat germ are very much alike in appearance. Commercial lecithin has a wide variety of uses. It is used to lubricate precision machines where oil needs to be spread thinly. It's also important in confectionery (candy making) and baking businesses for its natural homogenizing effect.

When Dad was associate editor of Macfadden's *Physical Culture Magazine* – he was sent on an expedition into China – soybean's original home. For thousands of years the Chinese have used soybeans. About 80% of their food is produced from soybeans in one form or another. Again Dad found many people who were living unbelievably long lives, like Zora Agha of Turkey. It was not unusual to find men and women from 125 to 135 years of age. Among these people, heart attacks, strokes, paralysis, coronary thrombosis and degenerative artery diseases were practically unknown! Eating soybeans in various forms meant they got large amounts of lecithin in their simple diet. The lecithin homogenized (dissolved) their dietary fats. Thus their level of blood-fat or blood cholesterol remained normal.

*There is a high concentration of lecithin in heart cells and in the sheathing around the brain, spinal cord and nerves. Lecithin comes in granules, liquid and capsules from the diversified, healthy soybean. **Lecithin is a natural fat emulsifier** and helps reduce larger, dangerous LDL cholesterol globules and elevates smaller, healthier HDL particles and also increases vital choline levels.*

Soybean Products for Healthy Heart & Nerves

We have been recommending the use of soybeans and its products to the health-conscious people of America since 1912. Lecithin – of which the soybean is the richest source – is not just important in the digestion of fats. The functioning of the nervous system and the glands are greatly aided by the phospholipids, one of the most important constituents of lecithin. That's why it's found in the nervous system and in every cell of the body. Nutritional Science teaches us that the nerves and cardiovascular system both require lecithin and the vitamin B-complex rich foods, see page 203-204.

Scientists have cited that breast cancer in Asian women is much lower than that in American women, largely due to the fact that Asian women consume a diet high in soy protein which contains isoflavones. These isoflavones are believed to lower blood cholesterol levels (page 118) which is vitally important for a healthy heart!

Carbohydrates: Starches & Sugars

Starches and sugars come under the classification, carbohydrates, in the FDA standard for food groups. These provide the principle source of food energy. Carbohydrates are needed as fuel for muscular work and physical activity. Excess sugars and starches that are not utilized as energy are transformed by the body chemistry into fat and stored in the least active body parts, causing obesity.

Carbohydrates originate in plants as sugars created by photosynthesis. Then they are formed into clusters as starches. Consumed by humans, they are broken down by the body's metabolism into a simple sugar – glucose – for use by the cells of the body. It is important that you eat only natural starches and sugars, and avoid those which are refined and depleted of vital elements (refined white flour, sugar and their refined products, etc.).

Natural starches and some natural sugars are found in all fresh fruits and vegetables, honey, pure maple syrup, sorghum, Stevia and blackstrap molasses, organic whole grains and their flours (wheat, oats, rye, etc.), beans, lentils and peas, organic brown rice and potatoes. In fact, all natural foods contain some carbohydrates.

Fats: Can Be Healthy or Unhealthy

Fat is also an important source of dietary energy. It has more than twice the energy value of the same amount of carbohydrates or protein. As already pointed out a certain amount of fat and even cholesterol is part of a healthy diet. Let us remind you that your fat intake should ideally consist of only unsaturated fats. The saturated fats in meat, eggs, poultry and dairy products often are best avoided or kept to a minimum. It is these saturated fats which can overload your body with excess cholesterol.

The Function of Fat in the Body

Our nerves, muscles and organs must be *cushioned* by a normal amount of fat. If we did not have a certain amount of fat in our *gluteus maximus* (the buttocks), for example, we would never be able to sit down because we would have to sit directly on our bones and muscles.

Those who wish to lose weight should reduce the *bad, saturated fat* content of their diet, and those who wish to gain should increase their *good, unsaturated fat* intake. But even when on a reducing diet, there should be some fat in your diet because it plays an important and essential role in your body's chemistry. Stored in the body, fat provides a source of heat and energy, while the accumulation of a certain amount of fat around the vital organs (such as the kidneys) gives great protection against cold and injury.

Fat also has a function to perform in the body's cells, for which special fats known as unsaturated fatty acids are needed in small amounts. Without these a roughness or scaliness of the skin would result. Fats have another all-important function: they carry the fat-soluble vitamins A, D, E and K through the body. As you can see, a certain amount of fat in the diet is necessary to a healthy functioning body. But it's the kind of fat that is most important! Unsaturated fat is best. Caution – it is wise to go light on the clogging saturated fats!

Dr. Dean Ornish has been able to reverse heart disease in more than 70% of his patients who follow, among other things, a low-fat vegetarian diet.

There are dozens of foods that contain almost NO bad fat and avocados and olives, fruits and vegetables have perfect ZERO fat!

Low-Fat Meals Help Cut Heart Disease Risk

A British research report by Dr. George Miller of Britain's Medical Research Council stated: *High fat meals make the blood more prone to clot within 6 to 7 hours after eating. Low fat meals can almost immediately reverse this condition. Most heart attacks occur in the early morning. One reason may be the overnight clotting effects of a high fat dinner. Researchers feel that by cutting fats from your diet, you may be able to add years to your life and cut the risk of heart disease!* Also University of Chicago research supports Dr. Dean Ornish and Dr. Miller's famous landmark statement that the healthiest meals for the heart are the low-fat, healthy vegetarian diets with ample fruits and vegetables.

Remember, meat-free and dairy-free is healthiest!

Organic Virgin Olive Oil Highly Recommended

Mother Nature has provided us with wonderful healthy oils which can be used in preparing foods, mayonnaise, salad dressings or for sautéing and marinating, etc. Virgin, cold-pressed olive oil has been used for centuries. Even Hippocrates used olive oil in his practice. Try Bragg's Organic Extra Virgin (first pressed) Olive Oil – it's the healthiest of oils!

Other healthy oils are cold-pressed safflower, sesame, sunflower and soybean oils. These oils can be used in salad dressings, recipes, baking, etc. We still use oils sparingly. They're healthy in polyunsaturated and unsaturated fatty acids. Please, don't use genetically engineered canola oil.

Another favorite oil of ours is organic unrefined flaxseed oil which is the richest source of omega-3 essential fatty acids (more than double that of fish oils). We also use hempseed oil. These two fragile oils must be kept cold, preferably in the freezer (they do not solidify) and they should not be heated. You can add them to foods after they have been cooked. We suggest you add 1 to 2 teaspoons daily of these oils to your diet, for the healthy omega fatty acids are vital to your bodily functions, especially the heart!

A Massachusetts Medical Society Study shows that using extra virgin olive oil lowers the need for blood pressure medication. The ones who used the olive oil reduced their blood pressure medication by 50%! Olive oil enhances health by lowering "bad" cholesterol without affecting "good" HDL. Try Bragg's Organic Extra Virgin Olive Oil. (See web: www.oliveoilsource.com or bragg.com)

Dr. Charles Attwood – Great Health Crusader

As a doctor, humanitarian, strong dedicated health crusader and a devoted pediatrician for over 40 years, and Fellow of the American Academy of Pediatrics, Dr. Charles Raymond Attwood fought many battles against mainstream medicine and big business to ensure the health of people everywhere, particularly children. He championed a low-fat vegetarian menu for children, was a strong health and nutrition activist and an associate of Dr. Benjamin Spock. One major battle occurred in 1996. As a member of the Center for Science in the Public Interest, Dr. Attwood led opposition to the giant Gerber Baby Food Company's practice of diluting its baby foods with water, sugar and starch. He won! Gerber stopped this 40 year crime against America's children. Now their foods are 100% fruits and vegetables. Other baby food companies then followed. See web: *vegsource.com*.

Dr. Attwood held high the banner advocating a low-fat, plant-based diet as the most healthy for youngsters. His highly praised 1995 book, *Low-fat Prescription for Kids* (available *Amazon.com*) makes a strong scientific argument for this diet. His research shows to avoid the leading causes of premature death later as adults: heart disease, stroke, cancers, diabetes, etc. it's important children follow his program.

116

Dr. Attwood's Tips for Low-Fat Shopping

- Spend most of your time in the produce department.
- Try new varieties of produce. Look at those with the most intense colors and remember organic is best!
- Don't forget about pasta made from whole-grains.
- Go straight for the whole-grain breads section.
- Buy unrefined, low-fat, sugarless, high-fiber cereals.
- When buying packaged, canned, frozen foods, read labels.
- Don't underestimate beans – whether dried, frozen or canned, they are delicious and healthy for you.
- Buy low- or no-fat healthy snacks – there's many choices. Careful, some are high in salt, sugar and calories.
- Replace milk and low-fat dairy products with soy, nut and rice milks, and soy and tofu cheeses, etc.

Seek out and choose whole foods, organic fruits, vegetables and organic whole grain cereals, breads, etc. rather than the commercial, canned, refined white flour and sugar products and other highly processed goods in the center aisles.

Fruits & Vegetables: Protective Foods

Remember that we told you that three-fifths of your diet should consist of organic, raw and lightly cooked vegetables and fresh fruits. These natural foods not only contribute isoflavins, vitamins and organic minerals to the diet, but they also add the bulk and moisture required for healthy elimination and smooth body functioning. They also help maintain the alkaline reserve of the body and add variety, color, flavor and texture to the diet.

Vegetables are virtually fat-free and contain no cholesterol! The ideal way to get the full amount of vitamins and minerals from organic vegetables is in their raw state, in fresh vegetable salads or as garnishes with meals. When cooking vegetables some vitamins and minerals may be lost.

What Are Live Foods?

Live foods are the living, vital foods for health and longevity and are perishable and some spoil quickly. America has been ignorant, foolish and almost idiotic in allowing various foods to be so refined that the vital and essential elements that Mother Nature gave them are refined out of them! They are buying and eating the depleted, devitalized mess that remains. This refining of foods is destroying America's health, hearts and bodies!

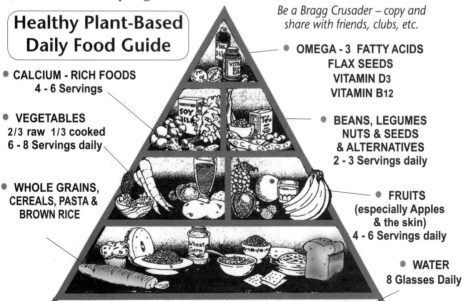

Healthy Plant-Based Daily Food Guide

Be a Bragg Crusader – copy and share with friends, clubs, etc.

- OMEGA - 3 FATTY ACIDS
  FLAX SEEDS
  VITAMIN D3
  VITAMIN B12

- CALCIUM - RICH FOODS
  4 - 6 Servings

- VEGETABLES
  2/3 raw 1/3 cooked
  6 - 8 Servings daily

- BEANS, LEGUMES
  NUTS & SEEDS
  & ALTERNATIVES
  2 - 3 Servings daily

- WHOLE GRAINS,
  CEREALS, PASTA &
  BROWN RICE

- FRUITS
  (especially Apples
  & the skin)
  4 - 6 Servings daily

- WATER
  8 Glasses Daily

8 Glasses Daily Purified/Distilled Water

Nature's Miracle Phytonutrients Help Prevent Cancer:

Make sure to get your daily dose of these naturally occurring, cancer-fighting super foods – phytonutrients that are abundant in apples, tomatoes, onions, garlic, beans, legumes, soybeans, cabbage, cauliflower, broccoli, citrus fruits, etc. The champions with the highest count of phytonutrients go to apples and tomatoes.

Class	Food Sources	Action
PHYTOESTROGEN ISOFLAVONES	Soy products, flaxseed, seeds & nuts, yams alfalfa & red clover sprouts, licorice root (not candy)	Helps block some cancers, & aids in menopausal symptoms and helps improve the memory
PHYTOSTEROLS	Plant oils, corn, soy, sesame, safflower, wheat, pumpkin	Blocks hormonal role in cancers, inhibits uptake of cholesterol from diet
SAPONINS	Yams, beets, beans, cabbage, nuts, soybeans	Helps prevent cancer cells from multiplying
TERPENES	Carrots, winter squash sweet potatoes, yams apples, cantaloupes	Antioxidants – protects DNA from free radical-induced damage
	Tomatoes & its sauces, tomato-based products	Helps block UVA & UVB and offers help to protect against cancers, prostate, etc.
	Spinach, kale, beet & turnip greens, cabbage	Protects eyes from macular degeneration
	Red chile peppers	Keeps carcinogens from binding to DNA
QUERCETIN (& FLAVONOIDS)	Apples, especially the skins, & red onions & green tea	Strong cancer fighter, protects heart & arteries. Reduces pain, allergy & asthma symptoms
	Citrus fruits (flavonoids)	Promotes protective enzymes
PHENOLS	Apples, fennel, parsley, carrots, alfalfa, cabbage	Helps prevent blood clotting & has some anticancer properties
	Cinnamon	Promotes healthy blood sugar and glucose metabolism
	Citrus fruits, broccoli, cabbage, cucumbers, green peppers, tomatoes	Antioxidants – flavonoids, block membrane receptor sites for certain hormones
	Apples, grape seeds	Strong antioxidants; fights germs & bacteria, strengthens immune system, veins & capillaries
	Grapes, especially skins	Antioxidant, antimutagen; promotes detoxification. Acts as carcinogen inhibitors
	Yellow & green squash	Antihepatoxic, antitumor
SULFUR COMPOUNDS	Onions & garlic, (fresh is always best) Red onions (our favorite) also contain Quercetin	Promotes liver enzymes, inhibits cholesterol synthesis, reduces triglycerides, lowers blood pressure, improves immune response, fights infections, germs & parasites

118

Raw Nuts and Seeds are Healthy Foods

Gary Null, a leading health activist writes in his book, *The Complete Guide to Sensible Eating*, that raw Nuts and Seeds are good sources of protein, minerals (especially magnesium), some B vitamins and unsaturated fatty acids (page 203). Nuts and Seed are delicious snack foods or used with other foods. There are few foods that are more highly packed with life force than raw seeds and nuts.

To make Nut Butters: Grind 1½ cups of raw unsalted nuts in a food processor or blender. Continue grinding nuts down until they're a thick, fudge-like paste. Then add sunflower or nut oil (start with 1 Tbsp and add more only if necessary), blend until smooth. Best kept refrigerated.

Flax and Chia are Seeds for Life

Flax Seeds are packed with omega-3, lignans and fiber, which are natural antioxidants. Omega-3 helps remove toxins and helps prevent heart disease (page 210). The lignans aid in preventing cancers and provide up to 700 times the amount of fiber found in legumes or whole grains. Fiber fights "bad" cholesterol and type 2 diabetes. Flaxseed improves conditions from cardiac and autoimmune functions to allergies and digestion. Other benefits include: healthier skin, hair and nails; 40-60% improvement in athletic performance; enhanced learning ability; and better brain development. Whole flaxseeds can be stored for months in airtight container in a cool, dark place, grind them in a coffee grinder as needed.

Chia Seeds are also rich in omega-3 fatty acids and antioxidants. Chia seeds provide fiber as well as calcium, phosphorus, magnesium, iron, niacin and zinc. They can slow down how fast our bodies convert carbohydrates into simple sugars, which may have great benefits for diabetics.

Chia seeds have a nutlike flavor. They are tasty, delicious and nutritious. You can sprinkle whole or ground chia seeds on cereal, yogurt, salads, soups and veggies. They can also be added to prepared infant formulas, baby foods and nutrition bars. You can also add them into flour when making baked goods such as cookies, muffins, etc.

Health Crusader Paul C. Bragg was the first to promote Chia and Flax Seeds.

Vitamin E-Rich Healthy Foods Are Important for Healthy Hearts

This is a list of healthy foods that contain the following notable amounts of precious vitamin E. Buy organic sources – they are best. Reference from National Institute of Health.

Food	Quantity	Vitamin E IU's
Apples	1 medium	1.21
Almonds	$^1/_4$ cup	13.37
Bananas	1 medium	0.40
Barley	$^1/_2$ cup	4.20
Beans, navy	$^1/_2$ cup	3.60
Bell Peppers	1 cup slices	0.94
Blueberries	1 cup	2.18
Broccoli	1 cup	1.12
Butter (salt-free)	6 tablespoons	2.40
Carrots	1 cup	0.45
Celery, green	$^1/_2$ cup	2.60
Corn oil	1 tablespoon	2.83
Eggs, fertile	2	2.62
Grapefruit	$^1/_2$	0.52
Kale	$^1/_2$ cup	8.00
Lettuce	6 leaves	0.50
Olive Oil (virgin)	1 tablespoon	2.38
Onions, raw	2 medium	0.26
Oranges	1 small	0.24
Papaya	1 medium	5.06
Peas, green	1 cup	4.00
Potatoes, white	1 medium	0.06
Potatoes, sweet	1 small	4.00
Rice, brown	1 cup cooked	2.40
Rye	$^1/_2$ cup	3.00
Soybean Oil	1 tablespoon	2.24
Sunflower Seeds, raw	1 oz.	8.94
Tomato	1 medium	1.01
Wheat Germ Oil	1 tablespoon	26.2

120

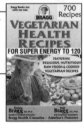
Recent revealing study of nurses whose daily vitamin E intake was 800 IU's and more, the nurses had a 36% amazing lower risk of heart attack and 23% lower risk of stroke.

Vitamin E & Raw Wheat Germ – Health Builders

Mother Nature invested raw wheat germ with one of the most valuable nutrients – vitamin E. And now it is coming to the aid of civilized man to help him regain the robust health he lost by eating devitalized foods. In the flour milling process, refining removes raw wheat germ to create white flour (staff of death). Millers realize wheat germ is fragile and goes rancid quickly. Refined foods have a long shelf life. Most Americans demand things they buy never spoil! That is why many American foods are refined and over 700 chemicals and poisons are used to preserve (embalm) them!

Famous Dr. Cureton of University of Illinois, who is recognized as one of the greatest living authorities on internal and external physical fitness, recommends raw wheat germ (little yellowish flakes), wheat germ oil and vitamin E capsules. They are especially useful in providing a great boost for athletes and others who desire to be in the highest state of physical fitness. Athletic coaches all over the world are following this advice to get the best performance from their athletes. In our opinion *raw wheat germ (vacuum packed), wheat germ oil and Vitamin E should be part of the nutritional program of everyone* – not just athletes! Vitamin E capsules are also recommended as the oil is more protected from rancidity.

Breakfast Should Be An Occasional Meal

On rare mornings when we eat breakfast, we have organic whole grain cereal, oatmeal or cornmeal, a sliced banana or fruit over cereal, with some honey, etc. and rice or soy milk. Make your own by combining 1 Tbsp of soy powder with $1/2$ glass water and $1/2$ tsp vanilla or pure maple syrup in a jar and shake. It's delicious and healthy!

A rich food source of vitamin E is cornmeal mush, made with organic stoneground yellow cornmeal (not the refined, dead, toxic GMO, degerminated variety found in supermarkets). On the next page is the Bragg family's favorite cornmeal recipe, plus a chart (page 120) for making sure you get vitamin E from these healthy foods you will enjoy!

The grains that are heart-healthy are organic brown rice, organic whole grain breads, cereals, and whole-wheat pastas. Also popcorn, organic corn is a whole grain. My favorite is air-popped and top with Bragg Liquid Aminos, Olive Oil and Nutritional Yeast (see recipe page 140). There's also bulgur, buckwheat groats, barley, millet, spelt, and quinoa. Quinoa is a complete protein and makes an ideal breakfast cereal.

Vitamin E – dynamic weapon against wrinkles & ageing. – Prevention Magazine

Patricia's Delicious Organic Cornmeal Mush

1 cup organic yellow cornmeal (coarse ground best)
2$\frac{1}{2}$ cups distilled water   2 Tbsp raisins or prunes (optional)

Moisten cornmeal with $\frac{1}{2}$ cup purified/distilled water. Boil remaining (2 cups) of water, then slowly add moistened cornmeal and raisins. When evenly thickened, turn heat to low and cook for 10 to 15 minutes. Serve hot. Top with honey, blackstrap molasses or 100% maple syrup, if desired (diabetics use Stevia). Top with sliced bananas or organic fresh fruit and try some soy, almond or rice milk.

NOTE: If you are serving to one or two people, there might be some mush left. Pour it into a flat pan, let it cool, and store in refrigerator. For breakfast – or even a main meal – slice and dip in egg batter and roll in wheat germ. Lightly heat in Bragg Organic Olive Oil and serve plain, hot, and top with honey, blackstrap molasses or maple syrup.

Soy Tofu Tasty Scramble

122

2 cups firm tofu, crumble   2 green onions, chop
2 tsps Bragg Organic Olive Oil   tomatoes, diced (optional)
$\frac{1}{8}$ tsp ground cumin $\frac{1}{2}$ tsp Bragg Liquid Aminos
$\frac{1}{4}$ tsp fresh garlic or powder   Bragg Sprinkle (24 herbs & spices)

In a wok, lightly sauté green onions in olive oil for 3 minutes, then add remaining ingredients (diced tomatoes or any fresh grated vegetables desired – keep stirring) cook 5-10 minutes longer. Tasty for breakfast or lunch. Serves 2 to 4.

Soy Tofu Whole Grain French Toast

$\frac{1}{2}$ lb tofu (soft) $\frac{1}{3}$ tsp cinnamon powder
$\frac{1}{4}$ tsp nutmeg   1 Tbsp honey

Blend tofu with enough water (distilled) to make a slightly runny batter. Dip the whole grain bread slices in batter and lightly sauté until brown in soy or olive oil or butter. Turn over, cook other side. Serve hot with honey or pure maple syrup. Serves 2. For variety, the Bragg family likes to have an occasional breakfast of steel-cut organic oats, cooked with raisins, prunes or sliced sun-dried apricots, topped with sliced bananas and 100% maple syrup. Yummy!

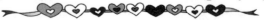

Add an ounce of love to everything you do.

Magnesium & Calcium Vital to Heart

Deficiencies of calcium and magnesium can produce all kinds of problems in the body – ranging from heart problems, dental decay and osteoporosis to muscular cramping, hyperactivity, muscular twitches, poor sleep patterns and also excessive frequency or uncontrolled urination patterns. Also, other mineral deficiencies or imbalances can cause health problems.

Therefore it's important to clean and detoxify the body by fasting and drinking only distilled, purified water and the juices of healthy organically grown vegetables and fruits. It's also important to provide the body with adequate sources of new minerals. This can be done by eating a diverse diet of organic vegetables that also includes kelp (see Bragg Sea Kelp, page 254) and other sea vegetables. Rice, soy and almond milks are good healthy alternatives instead of unhealthy cow's milk that causes mucus, etc. for babies, children and adults. See web: *notmilk.com*

Despite dietary sources as these, many adults and children living in so-called civilized cultures have low levels of essential minerals in their bodies. This is due to leeching caused by coffee, tea, cola, carbonated beverages and the ravages of long-term bad diets containing refined sugars, toxic aspartame and other sweets, as well as junk fast foods made from refined flours and foods containing high fat, high sugar, high salt and high cholesterol foods.

Additionally, the body's organ systems can be thrown out of balance by continued stress, toxins in our food, water and air, also by disease-produced injuries and by prenatal deficiencies arising from the mother's diet or lifestyle. The final result is that most people in our modern, fast-paced world are wise to take a natural multi-mineral and vitamin supplement (for extra insurance).

For optimal bone and cardiovascular health, nutritional experts for the past 40 years have urged those who take calcium to also supplement with magnesium, vitamin D and K. – Life Extension Magazine, Nov. 2010, www.lef.org.

The chemistry of food a person eats becomes his own body chemistry. Perhaps the most valuable result of all education is ability to inspire and make yourself do the thing you have to do, when it ought to be done, as it ought to be done, whether you like to do it or not! – Patricia Bragg, ND, PhD., Pioneer Health Crusader

Calcium is Important for a Fit Heart

Consider the shocking fact that 85% of Americans are deficient in calcium! Most people associate calcium with the teeth and bones, which is correct since a deficiency of this important mineral will lead to the deterioration of these hard tissues. Calcium is also very important for the nerves of the body. Many people suffer leg cramps due to a calcium deficiency. Calcium also plays an important role in the functioning of the heart. Calcium is a natural constituent of the material that causes the blood to clot. If we did not have calcium in our blood, we could prick a finger with a needle and bleed to death! Dad over 70 years ago, developed the first calcium supplement.

Every few minutes the heart is bathed by the calcium of the body chemistry. It is a crucial component in the activity of a healthy heart. Being the most powerful muscle in the entire body, the heart requires adequate calcium for its efficient functioning. Be good to your heart and maintain a good calcium balance. Study calcium chart next page.

124

Milk is Not a Good Source of Calcium

Nearly everyone has the idea that the problem of calcium deficiency will be solved if they just drink milk. This is not completely true. In the first place, practically all the milk in U.S. is pasteurized, which robs and greatly reduces the availability of milk's calcium (page 125 and web: *notmilk.com*).

Dr. Harold D. Lynch – famous author, researcher and physician – said recently **almost fanatic use of milk as a beverage has added more complications than benefits to child nutrition.** He further states **milk may often be a primary cause of poor nutrition in children!**

This might be due to the fact that proportionate amounts of Vitamins A and D and phosphorus must be present in the metabolism for the proper absorption and utilization of calcium by the body; another reason why proper nutrition and a balanced diet are so important!

Whole milk is a carrier of large amounts of saturated fat (cholesterol) and can lead to atherosclerosis. This food is just for cow's babies. It's wise for humans if they wish to maintain a healthy heart for a long life to eliminate milk.

Benefit From Natural Foods Rich in Calcium

There are some very fine sources of calcium other than milk. Scientists feel raw bonemeal is one of the best sources, as well as eggshell calcium, oyster shell calcium and bone marrow calcium. We prefer the calcium found in kale, spinach, corn, beans, veggies, soy tofu and sesame seeds. In fact, as Dr. Lynch and Dr. Neal Barnard point out, all natural foods contain appreciable amounts of calcium. This chart below shows foods that contain large amounts of calcium you should include in your diet.

Read 2 important books on milk & why best to avoid milk:

- *Mad Cows and Milk Gate* by Virgil Hulse M.D.
- *Milk, the Deadly Poison* by Robert Cohen

Both books on *amazon.com.* Also visit these websites:

- *www.notmilk.com* • *www.strongbones.org*
- *pcrm.org* (Physicians Committee for Responsible Medicine)

Calcium Content of Some Common Foods

Food Source	mgs	Food Source	mgs
Almonds, 1 oz	80	Kale, (raw/steamed)	180
Artichokes, (raw/steamed)	51	Kohlrabi, (raw/steamed)	40
Beans, (kidney, pinto, red)	89	Mustard greens, 1 cup	138
Beans, (great northern, navy)	128	Oatmeal, 1 cup	120
Beans, (white)	161	Orange, 1 large	96
Blackstrap molasses, 1 Tbsp	137	Prunes, 4 whole	45
Bok choy, (raw/steamed)	158	Raisins, 4 oz.	45
Broccoli, (raw/steamed)	178	Rhubarb, (cooked) 1 cup	105
Brussels sprouts, (raw/steamed)	56	Rutabaga, (raw/steamed)	72
Buckwheat pancake	99	Sesame seeds (unhulled) 1 oz	381
Cabbage, (raw/steamed)	50	Spinach (raw/steamed)	244
Cauliflower, (raw/steamed)	34	Soybeans,	73
Collards, (raw/steamed)	152	Soymilk, fortified	150
Corn tortilla	60	Tofu, firm	258
Cornbread, 1 piece	28	Turnip greens, 1 cup	198
Figs, (5 medium)	135	Whole wheat bread, 1 slice	17

Sources: *Back to Eden,* Jethro Kloss; *Health Nutrient Bible,* Lynne Sonberg; website: vrg.org/nutrition/calcium.htm, chart by Brenda Davis, R.D.

Many osteoporosis studies consistently conclude that vegetarians have stronger bones than meat-eaters. Many studies show that it's healthier to avoid meat and dairy products for optimum heart health.

It's strange that some men will drink and eat anything put before them, but check very carefully the oil they put in their car.

The Deadly Truth About Salt

For centuries, the expression *the salt of the earth* has been used as a catch-all phrase to describe something as good and essential. Yet nothing could be more wrong. That *harmless* product that you shake on top of your food every day may actually bury you before your time!

Consider these startling facts on salt:

1. **Salt is not a food!** There is no more justification for its culinary use than there is for potassium chloride, calcium chloride, barium chloride or any other harmful chemical that is used as a food seasoning.

2. **Salt cannot be digested, assimilated or utilized by the body.** Salt has no nutritional value! It has no vitamins! No organic minerals! No nutrients of any kind! Instead, it is positively harmful and can cause trouble in the kidneys, bladder, heart, arteries, veins, blood vessels and cause high blood pressure. Salt may waterlog tissues, causing water retention in the body.

3. **Salt may act as a heart poison.** It also increases the irritability of the nervous system and the body.

4. **Salt robs calcium from the body** and attacks the mucus lining throughout the gastrointestinal tract.

The Myth of the "Salt Lick"

Is a low-salt diet a nutritionally deficient diet? Don't we need plenty of salt in our diets to keep us in top physical condition? This is a popular notion, but is it true? People will tell you that animals will travel for miles to visit so-called *salt licks*. My father investigated the salt licks where wild forest animals congregated for miles around to lick the soil. The one chemical property all of these sites commonly known as *salt licks* had in common was *complete absence of sodium chloride (common salt)!* There was absolutely no organic or inorganic sodium at the salt licks! *But these soils had an abundance of organic minerals and nutrients which the animals naturally craved.*

It's a little known fact that about 80% of sodium we eat comes not from salt we add at the table or during cooking, but from processed, packaged foods.
– Tufts University Nutrition Letter • www.healthletter.tufts.edu

Salt Affects Your Blood Pressure & Weight

What causes high blood pressure? Medical Science recognizes many causes: tension, strains, stress, toxic substances such as cigarettes and gasoline, food additives, insecticide sprays, etc. and the side effects of drugs and industrial toxins are all suspect. What can you do to protect yourself from these injurious agents? You would do well to exclude as many of these harmful factors from your environment and life as soon as possible!

However, there is one cause of high blood pressure which can be easily avoided. *Sodium chloride (common table salt) is the major cause of high blood pressure!* Up to now, we have been talking about causing high blood pressure in the *normal* person. But how about the effects of salt on those millions suffering from our country's most prevalent and preventable ailment – excess weight? This is a prime area for research because obesity is known to be frequently accompanied by high blood pressure. Medical researchers proclaim a link between high blood pressure and salt intake in obesity.

Salt is Not Essential to Life

It is frequently claimed that salt is essential for life. However, there is no scientific basis to this belief. The truth is that entire primitive populations today use absolutely no salt and have never used it (most have no arthritis, cancer, etc.). If salt were essential to life, these people would have disappeared long ago. The proof salt is not needed is they are not only alive, but have better health than most Americans! Seems the *false necessity* of salt is mostly a money-making, harmful product.

Salt is Not Necessary to Combat Heat

There has been a great deal of propaganda in recent years about using salt in hot weather. The claim is made that the body loses a great deal of salt via perspiration and that this salt loss must be compensated for by consuming additional amounts of salt. Otherwise, according to this theory, great weakness and inability to continue normal activities will result. Hence factory workers are advised to take salt tablets in hot weather.

We have watched factory workers take these salt tablets, and have seen many of them become quite ill afterward. In fact, toxic reactions frequently follow the use of salt tablets. Vomiting and indigestion appear to be the 2 most common side effects and – as far as enabling one to stand the heat better is concerned – these dangerous salt tablets have no helping effect.

Death Valley Hike Proved Salt Dangerous

To prove definitely to my dad that he did not need salt during extremely hot weather, he went to Death Valley, California, one of the hottest spots in the entire world during July and August. On his first test he hired 10 husky young college athletes to make the hike in Death Valley from Furnace Creek Ranch to Stovepipe Wells, a distance of approximately 30 miles.

The boys had salt tablets and all the water they could drink . . . and a station wagon filled with plenty of food they wanted that contained salty foods like bread, buns, crackers, cheese, luncheon meats and hot dogs. They each ate, drank and took as many salt tablets as they desired. Dad had no salt, fasted during the 30 mile hike and drank water only. They began to hike on a sweltering July morning. The higher the sun rose, the hotter it became! Up went the heat until at noon it stood at 130 degrees – a dry, hot heat that seemed to want to melt and defeat these hikers!

The college boys gobbled the salt tablets and guzzled quarts of cool water. For lunch they drank cola drinks with ham and cheese sandwiches. They rested a half hour after lunch and then continued their rugged hike across the red hot blazing sands. Soon things were beginning to happen to those strong, husky college boys.

First, 3 of them got violently ill and threw up all they ate and drank for lunch. They got dizzy, turned deathly pale and weakness overcame them. They quit the hike immediately and were driven back to the Furnace Creek Ranch. The hike went on with 7 college athletes continuing.

The desire for salty foods is an acquired taste. Your tastebuds can be retrained to appreciate the true, natural flavors of foods. – Neal Barnard, M.D., *Food for Life.*

A laugh is just like sunshine. It freshens all the day. – Heart Warmers

Bragg - the Only Non-Salt User Finished Hike

As the hike progressed, the athletes drank large amounts of cold water and took more salt tablets. Then suddenly 5 of them got stomach cramps and became deathly ill. Up came the water and their lunch. These 5 had to be driven back. That left but 2 out of 10 hikers. It was now about 4 pm and the merciless sun beat down on them with great fury. Almost on the hour, the last remaining salt tablet-eating athletes collapsed and were rushed back for medical care.

That left only my dad on the test and he felt great! He was not full of salt tablets, nor food because he was on a fast. The college boys wanted cold water, but Dad drank only unchilled, distilled/purified water. He finished the 30 mile hike in good time and had no ill effects whatsoever! He camped out for the night. The next day he arose, and on purified/distilled water only, hiked another 30 miles back to the ranch without food or salt tablets. The doctors examined him and found him to be in excellent physical condition with no ill affects from the hot climate and the strenuous desert hike!

Break the Deadly Salt Habit – Start Now!

In our expeditions over the world we have met many primitive tribes in the tropics that use no salt. And while they are not bothered by the heat, salt-eating white people invariably complain about the hot weather. This seems to indicate that some commercial motive lies behind the *eat more salt in hot weather* campaign.

People undoubtedly would not add inorganic salt to their food if they were never taught to do so in the first place. *The taste for salt is an acquired one.* The craving for salt ceases a short time after it is eliminated from the diet. It is only during the first few weeks after the use of table salt is discontinued that it is really missed. After the initial period of abstinence there is little difficulty. In fact, many of our health students who have broken the deadly salt habit write us to say that now they cannot stand salted foods! When someone serves them salted foods, it gives them an abnormal thirst for liquids!! Their body wants to wash out the salt.

What Table Salt Does to Your Stomach

An important objection to table salt is the fact that it *interferes with the normal digestion of food.* Pepsin, an enzyme found in the hydrochloric acid of the stomach, is essential for the digestion of proteins. Only 50% as much pepsin is secreted as would otherwise be the case when salt is used. Obviously the digestion of protein foods will be incomplete or too slow under such conditions. The results are excessive putrefaction of protein, bloating, gas and digestive distress, which effects millions.

Sea Kelp is an Excellent Salt Substitute It's a Tasty, Healthy, Organic Sodium

Many outstanding heart specialists heartily endorse a no-salt diet. There are some excellent seasoning substitutes available to satisfy an acquired craving for salt. In the Bragg home we use Bragg Kelp, Sprinkle, herbs, garlic, vegetable seasonings and Bragg Liquid Aminos. In our opinion, sea kelp is an ideal salt substitute. It gives all foods – salads, vegetables, etc. – a tangy taste as Bragg Liquid Aminos does. Bragg Kelp Seasoning – sea kelp granules (rich in folate, calcium and magnesium to build new blood cells) and Bragg Sprinkle (24 herbs & spices) are available at health and grocery stores. Fresh and powdered garlic, lemon juice and Bragg Organic, Apple Cider Vinegar are excellent seasoners to add delicious flavors to foods.

Take a lesson from world famous French Chefs! The marvelous flavor of French dishes is achieved by the skillful use of garlic, onions, mushrooms, and great tasting herbs – not with salt! French cooking is called *rich* – but it's a richness of delicious natural taste. The best French Chefs use very little fat and most use no salt at all!

The American Heart Association says that daily sodium intake should be less than 2,400 milligrams per day, which is about 1¹/₄ teaspoons of sodium chloride (table salt –inorganic sodium). We recommend using NO table salt. Throwing away the salt shaker is a positive step towards living The Bragg Healthy Lifestyle! Get your natural organic sodium from natural healthy foods.

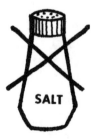

You will never improve your life until you change to live a 100% Healthy Lifestyle!

Natural Foods have Organic Sodium

Organic sodium is one of 16 minerals that are *required for perfect mineral balance* in the human body. Absorbable sodium is most plentiful organic mineral found in all fresh fruits and vegetables, *especially beets, celery and green beans.* Be assured that when you eat a balanced diet of plant-based natural foods you will receive sufficient organic sodium. Again, you must *put down that salt shaker and not pick it up again,* if you want a powerful, long-lasting heart!

Your Educated Taste Buds will Guide You

After you give up salt you will appreciate the natural flavor of foods. Dad was reared in the South where salt was used plentifully to season nearly all foods. His 260 taste buds were conditioned to the heavy taste of salt. At 16 he was a victim of tuberculosis. After three American Sanitariums and no improvement, his mother took him to a *Natural TB Sanitarium* in the Swiss Alps where they were against salt in the diet, something new to Dad! His health returned miraculously. (His sick body was cleansed and healed – nature's way for a miracle recovery.)

At first, Dad's taste buds rebelled. But no salt was permitted – so he re-educated his taste buds to a saltless diet. Any bad habit is difficult to overcome at first and the salt habit surely had Dad in its clutches, as salt, etc. has millions of Americans! But once his taste buds learned the difference, he started to taste and enjoy the real, natural, healthy flavors of food for the first time in his life!

Some health-minded people use *sea salt* rather than *table (land) salt.* There's little difference between these two! They are *both inorganic* and *loaded with sodium chloride!* Your 260 taste buds will guide you after you have discarded salt, for they will become very keen and sensitive and will reject salty foods. You will begin to enjoy tasting all the delicious flavors of natural foods.

According to studies most Americans consume "alarming" amounts of salt. Salt increases the risk of high blood pressure, a major cause of heart disease and stroke. Health officials estimate that about 80% of average American's salt intake occurs without them salting their food! It actually comes from salt in many packaged and processed foods, as well as restaurant and take-out meals. Stick to fresh organic fruits and vegetable and follow the Bragg Healthy Lilfestyle.

Eliminating Meat is Safer and Healthier!

Most uninformed nutritionists call meat the #1 source of protein. Those proteins coming from the vegetable kingdom are referred to as #2 proteins. This is a sad and terrible health mistake! It should be the other way around! Because in this day and age, almost all meat is laden with herbicides, fungicides, pesticides and other chemicals that are sprayed on or poured into the feed which these animals consume. They are also pumped full of growth hormones, antibiotics and all kinds of drugs to fatten them up and keep them from dying from extremely unhealthy conditions most of them live in! Many of them are forced-fed dead, groundup carcasses of other feed lot animals who, for a variety of sad reasons, didn't make it to the slaughterhouse.

The chemical reaction from fear is adrenaline! Fear is caused when a choke chain is around the neck of cattle to keep them in line. It's then shoved onto a conveyor belt and beheaded like those in front of them. Unused adrenaline is extremely toxic. Shocking most of the meat you consume is packed with this toxic substance!

Also, consider the fact that cattle, sheep, chickens, etc., are naturally vegetarians. When you eat them, you are just eating polluted vegetables. Why not skip all the waste and toxins and just eat healthy, organic vegetables?

It's a myth you have to eat meat to get your protein. Farm animals, especially horses, get protein! Horses are vegetarians and get protein from grains and grasses. You can get proteins (list on next page) you need from the large variety of whole grains, soy tofu, raw nuts, seeds, beans, fruits and vegetables that God put here for us.

Meat Has Toxic Uric Acid & Cholesterol

Meat is a major source of toxic uric acid and cholesterol, both harmful to your health! **If you insist on eating meat, it should be an organically fed source and not eaten more than 1 to 2 times weekly.** Fresh fish can be the least toxic of the flesh proteins. Beware, fish from polluted waters can be loaded with mercury, lead, cadmium, DDT and other toxins. If you are unsure of the waters the fish come from, don't risk eating it!

Excerpt from Bragg Vegetarian Recipe Book. Copy page and share with family, friends, etc.

Vegetarian Protein % Chart

LEGUMES %

Soybean Sprouts	54
Soybean Curd (tofu)	43
Soy flour	35
Soybeans	35
Broad Beans	32
Lentils	29
Split Peas	28
Kidney Beans	26
Navy Beans	26
Lima Beans	26
Garbanzo Beans	23

VEGETABLES %

Spirulina *(Plant Algae)*	60
Spinach	49
New Zealand Spinach	47
Watercress	46
Kale	45
Broccoli	45
Brussels Sprouts	44
Turnip Greens	43
Collards	43
Cauliflower	40
Mustard Greens	39
Mushrooms	38
Chinese Cabbage	34
Parsley	34
Lettuce	34
Green Peas	30
Zucchini	28
Green Beans	26
Cucumbers	24
Dandelion Greens	24
Green Pepper	22
Artichokes	22
Cabbage	22
Celery	21
Eggplant	21
Tomatoes	18
Onions	16
Beets	15
Pumpkin	12
Potatoes	11
Yams	8
Sweet Potatoes	6

GRAINS %

Wheat Germ	31
Rye	20
Wheat, hard red	17
Wild rice	16
Buckwheat	15
Oatmeal	15
Millet	12
Barley	11
Brown Rice	8

FRUITS %

Lemons	16
Honeydew Melon	10
Cantaloupe	9
Strawberry	8
Orange	8
Blackberry	8
Cherry	8
Apricot	8
Grape	8
Watermelon	8
Tangerine	7
Papaya	6
Peach	6
Pear	5
Banana	5
Grapefruit	5
Pineapple	3
Apple	1

NUTS AND SEEDS %

Pumpkin Seeds	21
Sunflower Seeds	17
Walnuts, black	13
Sesame Seeds	13
Almonds	12
Cashews	12
Macadamias	9

Data obtained from Nutritive Value of American Foods in Common Units, USDA Agriculture Handbook No. 456. Reprinted with author's permission, from *Diet for a New America* by John Robbins (Walpole, NH: Stillpoint Publishing)

Avoid shellfish – shrimp, lobster, crayfish! They are garbage-eating bottom-feeders and eat decaying scum, oil spills, etc. making them an unhealthy food choice.

Don't eat pork or pork products! Pigs are the only animals besides man that develops arteriosclerosis. This animal is so loaded with cholesterol that in cold winter weather, unprotected pigs can become stiff, very frozen solid and die. Also, pigs are often infected with a dangerous parasite which causes the disease trichinosis.

We feel that *meat and dairy products* are far more dangerous than they are healthy. Meats are high in visible fat, *invisible* fat, cholesterol and toxins from the animal. That's why we stress to meat eaters (if they must) not to have it more than 1 to 2 times a week and always trim off fat before cooking. Placing meat on a rack during cooking, baking or broiling helps drain off most of the fat and keeps it from soaking in its own unhealthy grease and drippings.

Don't eat greasy fried foods. The frying pan is the cradle of indigestion, heart disease and death! Those sputtering lumps of frying, sizzling fat are enemies of your heart and entire body! If you must eat meats, flavor with herbs, garlic, onions, mushrooms and Bragg Liquid Aminos, instead of fat-rich gravies. You can garnish meats with a variety of raw vegetables like watercress, parsley, celery, carrots, radishes, turnips, garlic, onions and bell peppers. Compared to meats, most fish is a better low fat protein! Buy freshly caught cold-water fish (salmon, halibut and mackerel) from unpolluted waters – it's healthier.

134

Poultry – chicken and turkey – the organically fed and hormone and drug free are safer animal proteins. Most poultry is commercially mass fed and heavily drugged with antibiotics and hormones. Guinea hen and squab are low in fat. But duck and goose are high in fat. Discard all poultry skins and giblets because they are high in fat.

Eggs. If you do eat eggs, limit to 2 or 3 per week. Remember, yolks contain high cholesterol fat. Fertile fresh eggs from free-range organic fed chickens are best.

Harvard University Medical School Researchers found that eating 2 to 3 eggs a week is unlikely to increase risk of heart disease. Plus, one egg has only 70 calories, is an excellent source of protein and essential nutrients including vitamins D, B12, riboflavin and folate. (We prefer the fertile, free range eggs.)

Almost every known food may cause some allergic reaction at times. Thus, foods used in elimination diets may cause allergic reactions in some individuals. Some are listed among the Most Common Food Allergies (see below). Since reaction to these foods is generally low, they are widely used in making test diets. By keeping a food journal and tracking your pulse rate after meals you will soon know your problem foods. Allergic foods cause pulse to go up. (Take base pulse before meals and then 30 minutes after meals. If it increases 8-10 beats per minute – check foods for allergies.) See web: *wrc.net/wrcnet_content/dietplans/cocoa_pulse_test.htm*

If your body has a reaction after eating a particular food, especially if it happens each time you eat that food, you may have an allergy. Some allergic reactions are: wheezing, sneezing, stuffy nose, nasal drip or mucus, dark circles, eye watering or waterbags under eyes, headaches, feeling light-headed or dizzy, fast heart beat, stomach or chest pains, diarrhea, extreme thirst, breaking out in a rash, swelling of extremities or stomach bloating, etc. (Read famous Dr. Arthur Coca's book, *The Pulse Test* – available on: *www.amazon.com*)

If you know what you're allergic to, you're lucky; if you don't, you better find out as fast as possible and eliminate all irritating foods from your diet. To reevaluate your daily life and have a health guide to your future, start a daily journal (8 $^1/_2$ x 11 notebook- enlarge and copy form on next page) of foods eaten, your pulse rate after meals and your reactions, moods, energy levels, weight, elimination and sleep patterns. You will discover the foods and situations causing problems. By charting your diet you will be amazed at the effects of eating certain foods. Dad kept a daily journal for over 70 years.

135

If you are hypersensitive to certain foods, you must omit them from your diet! There are hundreds of allergies and of course it's impossible here to take up each one. Many have allergies to milk, wheat, or some are allergic to all grains. Visit web: *foodallergy.org*. Your daily journal will help you discover and accurately pinpoint the foods and situations causing you problems. Start your journal today!

Most Common Food Allergies

- **MILK:** Butter, Cheese, Cottage Cheese, Ice Cream, Milk, Yogurt, etc.
- **CEREALS & GRAINS:** Wheat, Corn, Buckwheat, Oats, Rye
- **EGGS:** Cakes, Custards, Dressings, Mayonnaise, Noodles
- **FISH:** Shellfish, Crabs, Lobster, Shrimp, Shadroe
- **MEATS:** Bacon, Beef, Chicken, Pork, Sausage, Veal, Smoked Products
- **FRUITS:** Citrus Fruits, Melons, Strawberries
- **NUTS:** Peanuts, Pecans, Walnuts, chemically dried preserved nuts
- **MISCELLANEOUS:** Chocolate, Cocoa, Coffee, Black & Green (caffeine) Teas, Palm & Cottonseed Oils, MSG & Salt. Allergic reactions often caused by toxic pesticides, sprays, etc. on salad greens, vegetables & fruits, etc.

MY DAILY HEALTH JOURNAL

Today is:___/___/___

> **I have said my morning resolve and am ready to practice
> The Bragg Healthy Lifestyle today and every day.**

Yesterday I went to bed at: Today I arose at: Weight:

Today I practiced the No-Heavy Breakfast or No-Breakfast Plan: ☐ yes ☐ no

• For Breakfast I drank: Time:

  For Breakfast I ate:
                                                                    Time:

  Supplements:

• For Lunch I ate: Time:

  Supplements:

• For Dinner I ate: Time:

  Supplements:

• _____Glasses of Water I Drank during the Day

  List Snacks – Kind and When:

• I took part in these physical (walking, gym, etc.) activities today:

Grade each on scale of 1 to 10 (desired optimum health is 10).
• I rate my day for the following categories:

Previous Night's Sleep:	Stress/Anxiety:
Energy Level:	Elimination:
Physical Activity, Exercise:	Health:
Peacefulness:	Accomplishments:
Happiness:	Self-Esteem:

• General Comments, Reactions and To Do List:

Chapter 13

Eat to Live – Don't Live to Eat
Don't Overeat!

It's Harmful to Your Health to Overeat!

Second after second, minute after minute, hour after hour, day after day our faithful, loyal heart is working to keep us alive. In both our waking hours and during our sleep, our heart takes only a sixth of a second to rest between beats. The hardest work the heart has to do is right after an individual has eaten. The bigger the meal, the more work it has to do in pumping vast quantities of blood into the digestive tract.

> *Overeating puts more strain on the heart* than any other one thing! Many people load up on a ten-course dinner and soon afterward suffer a heart attack! Overeating is a dangerous, deadly habit that can lead to serious consequences! You should make it a habit to always get up from the table feeling that you could eat a little more.

 137

New studies done by the U.S. Center for Disease Control and Prevention, found that 66% of U.S. adults are overweight or obese and the rate is climbing yearly – it's an epidemic! Obesity is defined as anyone over 30% of their ideal body weight. This leads to high triglyceride levels which can cause diabetes and cardiovascular disease.

Remember, exercise is a major key factor in lowering your weight and helping keep the heart healthy and fit. Fact: only 20% of Americans exercise one hour weekly, yet they spend over 15 hours with TV and the web weekly.

Recent studies show people with large waistlines have shorter lifespans!

Sad Facts: *Many people go throughout life committing partial suicide – destroying their health, heart, youth, beauty, talents, energies and creative qualities. Indeed, to learn how to be good to oneself is often more difficult than to learn how to be good to others.* – Paul C. Bragg, ND, PhD.

Low-carb diets boost HDL "good" cholesterol and help with weight loss too!

Deep breathing is our connection to life, through the body and heart, leading us to a wholeness of being and giving us spirit for living life to its fullest. – S. Hainer

Current obesity studies show increases in all age groups. The biggest gain is in the 18 to 29 years old group at 12.1%, up from 7.1% back in 1991. American children (1 in 3) are more overweight now! Number of overweight children ages 6 to 17, has zoomed up since the 1960's. Overweight children are at high risks for adult on-set heart disease and diabetes! Teach your children healthy eating habits by being a healthy, trim, fit example for them!

It's Proven – Light Eaters Live Longer

My father's research and interviews with people who remained vigorous at ages over 100 years revealed that they ate sparingly, chewed thoroughly and never over-ate! Their diets were well-balanced with simple, natural foods. Scientific tests made on controlled animal feeding have also proven that light eaters live longer and in better health.

Always *give thanks first, (millions are starving), then eat slowly* and *chew food thoroughly*! Never eat in a hurry! Food bolted down causes trouble and it overworks the stomach and heart. Fast eating produces gas pressure on the heart and can cause heart attacks. If you don't have time to eat correctly, skip that meal! Fasting (see pages 147-154), skipping a meal occasionally is a good habit to develop.

Most eating habits form early in life from parents. To live long, feel youthful and have a powerful heart you must be able to avoid and rid yourself of bad eating habits, plus condition yourself to new, healthy eating habits and lifestyle!

A link was found between leptin, a protein hormone product of the obesity gene and risk for coronary heart disease. The study was conducted by the Imperial College School of Medicine in England. The obesity gene was cloned in 1994. Its product, leptin, acts as a signal to help the body decide when it has eaten enough food to feel full. The amount of leptin in the blood has been directly linked to body fat. This study is the first to associate leptin elevations in the blood with high blood pressure. Researchers measured leptin levels in 74 men. They found that the higher the level of leptin, the more likely the risk for heart disease. Measuring leptin may become a way of determining the risk of heart disease.

The longevity secret is eating & drinking intelligently. – Gaylord Hauser

Food and Product Summary

Today, many of our foods are highly processed or refined, robbing them of essential nutrients, vitamins, minerals and enzymes. Many also contain harmful, toxic and dangerous chemicals. The research findings and experience of top nutritionists, physicians and dentists have led to the discovery that devitalized foods are a major cause of poor health, illness, cancer and premature death. The enormous increase in the last 70 years of degenerative diseases such as heart disease, arthritis and dental decay substantiate this belief. Scientific research has shown that most of these afflictions can be prevented and that others, once established, can be arrested or even reversed through nutritional methods.

Enjoy Super Health with Natural Foods

1. **RAW FOODS:** Fresh fruits and raw vegetables organically grown are always best. Enjoy nutritious variety garden salads with raw vegetables, sprouts, raw nuts and seeds.

2. **VEGETABLES and PROTEINS:**
   a. Legumes, lentils, brown rice, soybeans, and all beans.
   b. Nuts and seeds, raw and unsalted.
   c. We prefer healthier vegetarian proteins. If you must have animal protein, then be sure it's hormone–free, and organically fed and no more than 1 or 2 times a week.
   d. Dairy products – fertile range-free eggs (*not over 3-4 weekly*), unprocessed hard cheese and feta goat's cheese. We choose not to use dairy products. Try the healthier non-dairy soy, rice, nut, and almond milks and soy cheeses, delicious soy yogurt and soy and rice ice cream.

3. **FRUITS and VEGETABLES:** Organically grown is always best, grown without use of poisonous sprays and toxic chemical fertilizers. Urge markets to stock organic produce! Steam, bake, sauté and wok vegetables as short a time as possible to retain best nutritional content, flavor and use raw veggies in salads, sandwiches, etc. Also enjoy fresh juices.

4. **100% WHOLE GRAIN CEREALS, BREADS and FLOURS:** They contain important B-Complex vitamins, vitamin E, minerals, fiber and the important unsaturated fatty acids.

5. **COLD or EXPELLER-PRESSED VEGETABLE OILS:** Bragg Organic Extra Virgin Olive Oil (is best), soy, sunflower, flax and sesame oils are excellent sources of healthy, essential, unsaturated fatty acids. We still use oils sparingly.

HEALTHY BEVERAGES
Fresh Juices, Herb Teas & Energy Drinks

These freshly squeezed organic vegetable and fruit juices are important to The Bragg Healthy Lifestyle. It's not wise to drink beverages with your main meals, as it dilutes the digestive juices. But it's great during the day to have a glass of freshly squeezed orange, grapefruit, vegetable juice, Bragg Vinegar ACV Drink, herb tea or try hot cup Bragg Liquid Aminos Broth ($^1/_2$ to 1 tsp. Bragg Liquid Aminos in cup of hot distilled water) – these are all ideal pick-me-up beverages.

Bragg Apple Cider Vinegar Cocktail – Mix 1 to 2 tsps. Bragg Organic ACV and (*optional*) to taste raw honey, agave nectar or pure maple syrup in 8 oz. of distilled or purified water. Take glass upon arising, hour before lunch and dinner (*if diabetic, to sweeten use 2 stevia drops*). Bragg Organic ACV drinks now available in 4 fruit flavors, see page 256.

Delicious Hot or Cold Cider Drink – Add 2 to 3 cinnamon sticks and 4 cloves to water and boil. Steep 20 minutes or more. Before serving add Bragg Vinegar and sweetener to taste (*Re-use cinnamon sticks & cloves*).

Bragg Favorite Juice Cocktail – This drink consists of all raw vegetables (please remember organic is best) which we prepare in our vegetable juicer: carrots, celery, beets, cabbage, tomatoes, watercress and parsley, etc. The great purifier, garlic we enjoy, but it's optional.

Bragg Favorite Healthy Energy Smoothie – After morning stretch and exercises we often enjoy this drink instead of fruit. It's delicious and powerfully nutritious as a meal anytime: lunch, dinner or take in thermos to work, school, sports, gym, hiking, and to park or freeze for popsicles.

Bragg Healthy Energy Smoothie

Prepare following in blender, add frozen juice cube if desired colder; Choice of: freshly squeezed orange or grapefruit juice; carrot and greens juice; unsweetened pineapple juice; or $1^1/_2$ - 2 cups purified or distilled water with:

2 tsps spirulina or green powder	1 to 2 bananas, ripe
$^1/_3$ tsp Bragg Nutritional Yeast	or fresh fruit in season
2 dates or prunes, pitted (optional)	1-2 tsps almond or nut butter
1 "Emergen-C" Vitamin C packet	$^1/_2$ tsp lecithin granules
1 tsp protein powder	1 tsp raw honey (optional)
$^1/_2$ tsp flax seed oil or grind seeds	$^1/_2$ tsp rice or oat bran

Optional: 4 apricots (sundried, unsulphured) soak in jar overnight in purified/distilled water or unsweetened pineapple juice. We soak enough to last for several days. Keep refrigerated. In summer you can add organic fresh fruit: peaches, papaya, blueberries, strawberries, all berries, apricots, etc. instead of banana. In winter, add apples, kiwi, oranges, tangelos, persimmons or pears, and if fresh is unavailable, try sugar-free, frozen organic fruits. Serves 1 to 2.

Patricia's Delicious Health Popcorn

Use freshly popped organic popcorn (use air popper). Try Bragg Organic Olive Oil or flax seed oil or melted salt-free butter over popcorn and add several sprays of Bragg Liquid Aminos and Bragg Apple Cider Vinegar – Yes, it's delicious! Now sprinkle with Bragg Nutritional Yeast Seasoning and Bragg Sprinkle (24 herbs & spices). For a variety try a pinch of cayenne pepper, mustard powder or fresh crushed garlic to oil mixture. Serve instead of breads!

Bragg Lentil & Brown Rice Casserole, Burgers or Soup
Jack LaLanne's Favorite Recipe

14 oz pkg lentils, uncooked
4 - 6 carrots, chop 1" rounds
3 celery stalks, chop, (optional)
2 onions, chop, (optional)
5-6 cups, distilled /purified water

$1^1/_2$ cups brown organic rice, uncooked
4 garlic cloves, chop, (optional)
1 tsp Bragg Liquid Aminos
$1/_4$ tsp Bragg Sprinkle (24 Herbs & Spices)
2 tsps Bragg Organic Virgin Olive Oil

Wash & drain lentils & rice. Place grains in large stainless steel pot. Add water, bring to boil, reduce heat, then add vegetables & seasonings to grains and simmer for 30 minutes. If desired, last 5 minutes add fresh or canned (salt-free) tomatoes before serving. For delicious garnish add spray of Bragg Aminos, minced parsley & Bragg Nutritional Yeast Seasoning. Mash or blend for burgers. For soup, add more water. Serves 4 to 6.

Bragg Raw Organic Vegetable Health Salad

2 stalks celery, chop
1 bell pepper & seeds, dice
$1/_2$ cucumber, slice
2 carrots, grate
1 raw beet, grate
1 cup green cabbage, chop

$1/_2$ cup red cabbage, chop
$1/_2$ cup alfalfa or sunflower sprouts
2 spring onions & green tops, chop
1 turnip, grate
1 avocado (ripe)
3 tomatoes, medium size

For variety add organic raw zucchini, sugar peas, mushrooms, broccoli, cauliflower, (try black olives & pasta). Chop, slice or grate vegetables fine to medium for variety in size. Mix vegetables & serve on bed of lettuce, spinach, watercress or chopped cabbage. Dice avocado and tomato and serve on side as a dressing. Serve choice of fresh squeezed lemon, orange or dressing separately. Chill salad plates before serving. **It's best to always eat salad first before hot dishes.** Serves 3 to 5.

Bragg Health Salad Dressing

$1/_2$ cup Bragg Organic Apple Cider Vinegar
1-2 tsps organic raw honey
$1/_2$ tsp Bragg Liquid Aminos
1-2 cloves garlic, minced
$1/_3$ cup Bragg Organic Olive Oil, or blend with safflower, soy, sesame or flax oil
1 Tbsp fresh herbs, minced or pinch of Bragg Sprinkle (24 herbs & spices)

Blend ingredients in blender or jar. Refrigerate in covered jar.

FOR DELICIOUS HERBAL VINEGAR: In quart jar add $1/_3$ cup tightly packed, crushed fresh sweet basil, tarragon, dill, oregano, or any fresh herbs desired, combined or singly. (If *dried* herbs, use 1-2 tsps herbs.) Now cover to top with Bragg Organic Apple Cider Vinegar and store two weeks in warm place, and then strain and refrigerate.

Honey – Celery Seed Vinaigrette

$1/_4$ tsp dry mustard
$1/_4$ tsp Bragg Liquid Aminos
$1/_4$ tsp paprika or to taste
2-3 Tbsps raw honey or to taste

1 cup Bragg Organic Apple Cider Vinegar
$1/_2$ cup Bragg Organic Extra Virgin Olive Oil
$1/_2$ small onion, minced
$1/_3$ tsp celery seed (or vary amount to taste)

Blend ingredients in blender or jar. Refrigerate in covered jar.

Avoid These Processed, Refined, Harmful Foods

Once you realize the harm caused to your body by unhealthy refined, chemicalized, deficient foods, you'll want to eliminate these "killer" foods. Also avoid microwaved foods! Follow The Bragg Healthy Lifestyle to provide the basic, healthy nourishment to maintain your health.

• Refined sugar, artificial sweeteners (toxic aspartame) or their products such as jams, jellies, preserves, marmalades, yogurts, ice cream, sherbets, Jello, cake, candy, cookies, all chewing gum, colas & diet drinks, pies, pastries, & all sugared fruit juices & fruits canned in sugar syrup. **(Health Stores have delicious healthy replacements, such as Stevia, raw honey, 100% maple syrup, & agave nectar, so seek & buy the best.)**

• White flour products such as white bread, wheat-white bread, enriched flours, rye bread that has white flour in it, dumplings, biscuits, buns, gravy, pasta, pancakes, waffles, soda crackers, pizza, ravioli, pies, pastries, cakes, cookies, prepared and commercial puddings and ready-mix bakery products. Most are made with dangerous (oxy-cholesterol) powdered milk and powdered eggs. **(Health Stores have huge variety of 100% whole grain organic products, delicious breads, crackers, pastas, desserts, etc.)**

• Salted foods, such as corn chips, potato chips, pretzels, crackers and nuts.

• Refined white rices and pearled barley. • Fried fast foods. • Indian ghee.

• Refined, sugared (also aspartame) dry processed cereals – cornflakes, etc.

• Foods that contain olestra, palm and cottonseed oil. These oils are not fit for human consumption and should be totally avoided .

• Peanuts and peanut butter that contain hydrogenated, hardened oils and any peanut mold and all molds that can cause allergies.

• Margarine – combines heart-deadly trans-fatty acids and saturated fats.

• Saturated fats and hydrogenated oils – enemies that clog the arteries.

• Coffee, decaffeinated coffee, caffeinated tea and all alcoholic beverages. Also all caffeinated and sugared water-juices, all cola and soft drinks.

• Fresh pork and products. • Fried, fatty, greasy meats. • Irradiated GMO foods.

• Smoked meats, such as ham, bacon, sausage and smoked fish.

• Luncheon meats, hot dogs, salami, bologna, corned beef, pastrami and packaged meats containing dangerous sodium nitrate or nitrite.

• Dried fruits containing sulphur dioxide – a toxic preservative.

• Don't eat chickens or turkeys that have been injected with hormones or fed with commercial poultry feed containing any drugs or toxins.

• Canned soups - read labels for sugar, salt, starch, flour and preservatives.

• Foods containing benzoate of soda, salt, sugar, cream of tartar and any additives, drugs, preservatives; irradiated and genetically engineered foods.

• Day-old cooked vegetables, potatoes and pre-mixed, wilted lifeless salads.

• All commercial vinegars: pasteurized, filtered, distilled, white, malt and synthetic vinegars are dead vinegars! (*We use only our Bragg Organic Raw, unfiltered Apple Cider Vinegar with the "Mother Enzyme" as used in olden times.*)

You need to learn not only what to leave out of your diet, but also, as importantly, what you should put into it. You will find that you can nourish your body without sacrificing meal-time enjoyment once you understand the basic health principles of proper nourishment. This knowledge will show you the elements your body needs to build, develop and live healthily as it was meant to do naturally. Combinations of healthful foods packed with vital nutrients are abundant worldwide.

The first step, of course, is to get into *the habit of eating for health*. Such a habit is not difficult to form. Although the instinctive sense of food selection has been submerged with all the advertising of the popular fast, junk foods, etc. You have to be strong minded! Like any other ability or skill, a healthy lifestyle must be kept constantly in practice or its powers will deteriorate. Only by exercising this natural health instinct and desire can we revive and strengthen our health.

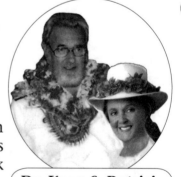

Dr. Koop & Patricia
Hawaii Health Conference

(143)

Bad Nutrition – #1 Cause of Sickness
"Diet-related diseases account for 68% of all deaths."
– Dr. C. Everett Koop

America's former Surgeon General and our friend, said this in his famous 1988 landmark report on nutrition and health in America. People don't die of infectious conditions as such, but of malnutrition that allows the germs to get a foothold in sickly bodies. Also, bad nutrition is usually the cause of non-infectious, fatal or degenerative conditions. When the body has its full nutrition quota of vitamin and minerals, including potassium, it's almost impossible for germs to get a foothold in a healthy, powerful bloodstream and tissues!

What a person eats and drinks becomes his own body chemistry. – Paul Bragg

Good health and good sense are two of life's greatest blessings. – P. Syrus

Proper Nutrition for Rejuvenation & Fitness

Degenerative diseases stem from breakdowns within the body, not attacks from outside, although the latter may occur secondarily as a result of weakened defenses. Since degenerative diseases arise within our bodies because of some lack of a vital element or substances, our safest course is to reinforce our defenses with those nutrients which will build our powers of resistance. *Your body is like a fortress.* Although people may look alike on the *outside, the inside* determines their strengths and weaknesses. Well-marshaled forces within a fortress can repel an enemy, while poorly organized forces will succumb. Let's build our inner strength so we will be impervious to all deadly enemies of the body!

Don't Clog Arteries with Fats & Bad Foods

As poisons accumulate in your body, it becomes impossible to have smooth, flexible arteries through which oxygen-enriched blood can flow freely. The toxins, tars and chemicals from unhealthy foods, saturated fats and tobacco, caffeine teas, coffee and colas, leave a poisonous residue on the arteries. Not only do these fats and poisons clog your arteries, but the tobacco, coffee, teas, cola, and alcohol drinks are also unhealthy stimulants to the heart. The heart has a natural rhythm which it can maintain indefinitely under most normal conditions. When you use these harsh stimulants, you actually whip and beat your heart into unnatural activity causing it to be overworked, overstressed and this is unhealthy!

Beware of "Killer" Foods

If drink can kill — so can food! Don't dig your grave with your knife and fork! To have a heart that is fit, your blood chemistry must be healthy and balanced. The 5 to 6 quarts of blood in your body must have all of the *60 nutrients that build and maintain a powerful, fit heart.*

Years ago people did not need to know what to leave out of their diet. That was because the only foods that they had to eat were those produced by Mother Nature. These foods were not robbed of their natural elements like today's foods that are processed and preserved and embalmed by the greedy food industry to stay fresh.

No One Need Suffer Heartburn

If the way to a person's heart is through their stomach, then heartburn (*acid indigestion*) is the end of the romance. Heartburn is a much misunderstood condition that has been written about since Roman times. *First*, it has little to do with the heart. *Second*, it has little to do with spicy or acidic foods. It is caused when the stomach's contents back up into the lower throat (the esophagus). These powerful stomach acids, which are stronger and more acidic than even the spiciest of foods, burn the sensitive walls lining the esophagus.

Apple Cider Vinegar Relieves Heartburn

It is vitally important that you don't join the millions of Americans who regularly take a variety of antacids, seltzers, etc. These over-the-counter medications neutralize stomach acids which only further throws off a digestive process already out of balance. You must reduce the amount of fat in your diet because fatty foods cause stomach acids to back up into the esophagus. Also, don't dilute your precious digestive juices by drinking water, juices and herbal teas with your meals. Make it a habit to enjoy beverages between (not during) meals.

When it comes to good digestion, you must practice good posture – sit up tall and straight, lifting up your chest with your shoulders slightly back. This will keep your esophagus, stomach and intestines properly aligned and will not crowd your vital machinery. Most importantly remember your stomach has no teeth! You must chew each and every mouthful of food slowly and thoroughly to a pulp (Fletcherizing) that slides down easily. This helps insure a painless, healthy digestion of your meals.

Dr. Gabriel Cousins, author of *Conscious Eating*, treats his patients heartburn and Gerds with simple sips of $1/3$ teaspoon of Bragg's Organic Apple Cider Vinegar before meals. Plus, do enjoy the Bragg's famous healthy delicious Vinegar Drink 3 times daily (pages 140, 248 and 256).

Dr. Cousins says: *Bragg's Organic Apple Cider Vinegar with the 'Mother' is the #1 food I recommend to maintain the body's acid-alkaline balance and to stop Gerds.*

Olive Oil – Mediterranean's Tasty Heart Treat

Olives have been used for centuries. Not only are they eaten and used on foods and in cooking, but olive oil is used for ointments, body lotion and in many other ways. In 400 B.C. Hippocrates, the Greek physician (the father of medicine) wrote about the great curative properties of olive oil he called the great therapeutic. He also told of the powerful cleansing and healing properties of apple cider vinegar (pages 140, 248 and 256). *www.oliveoilsource.com*

The words of Hippocrates still hold true today. In 1994, the Lyon Diet Heart Study wanted to find out why the people of the Mediterranean region had much less heart disease than Americans and Northern Europeans. The answer was found in the characteristic diet of the region. Spanish, Italians and Greeks share a diet that is much lower in saturated fats than the diet of those regions with high rates of heart disease. The dietary fat of the Mediterranean residents is primarily olive oil.

The Lyon Diet Heart Study (For more on this study see web: *www.AmericanHeart.org*) and other European research has found that olive oil offers great cardiovascular rewards. After 2 years, people who decreased their fat intake and ate most of the remaining fat in the form of olive oil had a 76% decrease in new heart trouble. The greatest reduction was angina pains and non-fatal heart attacks.

Olive oil beneficially influences cardiovascular health by reducing cholesterol levels. It helps protect and strengthen the digestive system by providing the body with *polyphenols* (powerful antioxidant compounds). Don't let this delicious, healthy gift of Mother Nature pass you by! Make Bragg Organic Olive Oil a part of your diet. Dr. Julian Whitaker says it's the best for the heart.

Nutritionist have been studying the Mediterranean diet for the last 20 years and have found that the residents have a very low incidence of heart disease. With the recent discovery of "good" cholesterol (HDL), scientists have begun to understand why people from the Mediterranean area have a very healthy cholesterol balance, with their high consumption of olive oil. This is because olive oil helps stimulate body's production of "good" HDL, that helps the body limit the buildup of substances that block arteries, that cause heart disease.
– Martha Rose Shulman, *Mediterranean Light*

For where your treasure is, there will your heart be also. – Matthew 6:21

Chapter 14

Doctor Fasting

Fasting – the Perfect Heart-Rester

If you are vitally interested in having a strong heart, you must skip 1 or 2 meals a week or even better, fast for one whole day out of 7. What a wonderful rest the hard-working heart receives when you take a day or 2 of total abstinence from all food! Just drink 8-10 glasses distilled water daily (add vinegar to 3, page 140). If you need something warm, have herb tea – mint, alfalfa, anise seed, etc. or Bragg Vinegar Drink. You may add 1/2 tsp honey to herb tea if desired. During water fast partake of no juices or food.

A Story of Successful Fasting

We have thousands of letters in our files from health students all over the world, who have had remarkable recoveries with fasting. One of these students had a serious heart attack at 55 years of age. She was flat on her back in bed for 8 weeks. When she finally got up she was a pitiful sight – pale, haggard and weak. She was thoroughly discouraged since she had been told that she did not have long to live.

Then she got hold of our Bragg book *The Miracle of Fasting* and started to fast 1 day each week. After a few months she fasted for 3 or 4 days each month. Then she went on a 7 day fast. Great cleansing and healing took place in her body because of her fasting and living The Bragg Healthy Lifestyle. NOTE: The Bragg Book *The Miracle of Fasting* is a complete and instructive program on the Science of Fasting. See pages 245-247 of this book for the complete Bragg Self-Health book list.

Banish All of Your Fears About Fasting!

The average person has a preconceived notion that if they skip a few meals or fast for a few days, dangerous things will happen to their body. Nothing is farther from the truth! My father and I have fasted for as many as 30 days straight – and felt stronger on the 30th day than when the fast started! Caution! We don't advise our students to go on long fasts unless needed and supervised by a health professional. Inquire for good contacts at health stores, health clubs, etc. or check *spafinder.com.*

Nothing will give the body more energy and vitality than fasting. Fasting also strengthens the body's digestive system and heart. Forget your fears! Fasting cleanses the internal body. Try a short fast to demonstrate to yourself the miracles fasting can accomplish in your life!

Here's our personal fasting program for you: We fast on Mondays. During this time we drink 8 to 10 glasses of distilled water, 3 with Bragg Vinegar (page 140). This gives our digestive and elimination systems a complete rest. We then eat on Tuesday. This rest from food takes a great load off of the hard-working heart and digestive system and helps keep body cleaner and healthier.

Several times yearly we take a longer *super* fast. We usually prefer a distilled water fast for 7 to 10 days. This works wonders in keeping us fit, trim and healthy (page 154)! The Hollywood Stars love juice fasting to detox (page 150).

Cleansing the Heart Pump and Pipes

If our *pipes* and great *pump* are clogged and corroded with debris and toxic poison we cannot be physically fit! Therefore, it is necessary from time to time to give the *pipes* and the *pump* of the body a thorough cleansing. This should be done by fasting once every week – for this 1 day will have beneficial effects. It will shake the toxins loose from the tissues, stimulate circulation and get rid of foreign matter that has become encrusted in the heart and blood vessels.

You should follow this cleansing program at least 1 day a week. Then in time you will have enough fortitude to fast for 3 days straight – you will be amazed at the results! If you have any reactions during this cleansing program – such as headaches, excessive gas or feeling of weakness – just remember that this is what we call a *healing crisis.* These symptoms will fade away as the toxins pass through your elimination system.

Fasting is the greatest remedy – the physician within!
– Paracelsus, 15th century physician, established role of chemistry in medicine.

Along with a weekly 24 hour fast, daily tongue brushing and spoon scraping during oral hygiene (brushing, flossing) is a wise health practice, as your body is continually cleansing from your anus to your tongue. – Patricia Bragg, ND, PhD.

Flushing Poisons from Your Body's "Pipes"

While on this Cleansing Program, drink at least a half a gallon of distilled (purified) water daily – that is free of toxic chemicals. The night before you start this regime take 1 to 2 quarts of distilled water and add to it 2 whole carrots cut into pieces, 3 diced stalks of celery (leaves and all), 1 handful of chopped parsley and 1 beet cut up fine. *Soak this mixture overnight.* After it has soaked 10 hours or more, strain the vegetable-distilled water and discard the vegetables (great for compost). Use this water, in which the vegetables have been soaked, as part of your drinking water during first day for your cleansing.

On arising have Bragg Vinegar Cocktail (page 140) and hour later eat an apple and a few sun-dried figs or dates, 1 glass of prune juice (add 1 tsp mixed oat bran and psyllium).

At 10 a.m. eat some fresh fruit (oranges, grapefruit, bananas, apples, pears, grapes, etc.) and drink cup herbal tea, greens drink or Bragg Liquid Aminos broth (1 tsp. to 1 cup water). If you take supplements, do so now.

At 12 noon enjoy tossed green salad of sliced cabbage with grated carrots and beets, chopped green onion, celery, bell pepper, parsley, raw spinach, watercress, tomato and 2 cloves finely chopped garlic. Eat this salad with the salad dressing recipes found on page 141 or buy the Bragg Ginger Sesame Dressing or the Bragg Healthy Vinaigrette Dressing available at Health Stores. You may also have a lightly cooked vegetable (low in natural sugar) such as string beans, squash or any green leafy vegetables, kale, etc.

At 3 p.m. eat fresh fruit, such as apples, grapes, pears, bananas or a few dried fruits as dates, figs, prunes, etc. and a cup of hot distilled water with 1 tsp of Bragg Aminos.

At 6 p.m. supper, tossed vegetable/green salad as lunch and bowl of lightly steamed greens (kale, mustard or turnip greens, beet tops, spinach, etc.) cooked with chopped onions, 2 garlic cloves and before serving add Tbsp. Organic Olive Oil and sprinkle with Bragg Nutritional Yeast. After meal you may take your evening supplements.

Flaxseed Cleanse – optional – *may take once daily:*
Soak Tbsp. flaxseeds (1 hour) in glass distilled water, vinegar drink or cup herb tea. Stir, drink hour after dinner.

Juice Fast – Introduction to Water Fast

Fasting has been rediscovered, through juice fasting, as a simple, easy means of cleansing and restoring health and vitality. To fast (abstain from food) comes from the Old English word *fasten* or *to hold firm.* It's a means to commit oneself to the task of finding inner strength through body, mind and soul cleansing. Throughout history the world's greatest philosophers and sages – including Socrates, Plato, Buddha, Gandhi and our Creator Jesus – practiced fasting and preached its benefits!

Juice bars are springing up everywhere and juice fasting has become *in* with the theatrical crowd in Hollywood, New York and London. The number of Stars who believe in the power and effectiveness of juice and water fasting is growing. A partial list includes: Steven Spielberg, Barbra Streisand, Kim Basinger, Alec Baldwin, Daryl Hannah, Christie Brinkley, Dolly Parton and Donna Karan. They say fasting helps balance their lives physically, mentally, spiritually and emotionally. Although we feel a water fast is best, an introductory liquid juice fast can offer people an ideal opportunity to give their intestinal systems a restful, cleansing relief from the high fat, high sugar, high salt and high protein fast foods too many Americans unhealthfully exist on!

Organic, raw, live fruit and vegetable juices can be purchased fresh from Health Stores. You can also prepare these healthy juices yourself using a good home juicer. When juice fasting, it's best to dilute juice with 1/3 distilled water. The list on the next page gives you many delicious combination ideas. With any vegetable and tomato combinations try adding a dash of Bragg Liquid Aminos, herbs or, on non-fast days, even some green powder (barley, chlorella, spirulina, etc.) to create a delicious, nutritious, powerful health drink. When using herbs in these drinks, use 1 to 2 fresh leaves or pinch of Bragg Sprinkle (24 herbs & spices) or Bragg Kelp (seaweed), rich in protein, iodine and iron is delicious with vegetable juices.

Fasting is an effective and safe method of detoxifying the body – a technique used for centuries for healing. Fast regularly one day a week and help the body cleanse and heal itself to stay well. When a cold or illness is coming on, or even depression – it's best to fast! Bragg Books were my conversion to the healthy way.
– James Balch, M.D. Co-Author of Prescription for Nutritional Healing

Delicious, Powerful Juice Combinations:

1. Beet, celery, alfalfa sprouts
2. Cabbage, celery and apple
3. Cabbage, cucumber, celery, tomato, spinach and basil
4. Tomato, carrot and celery
5. Carrot, celery, watercress, garlic and wheatgrass
6. Grapefruit, orange and lemon
7. Beet, parsley, celery, carrot, mustard greens, cabbage, garlic
8. Beet, celery, kelp and carrot
9. Cucumber, carrot and celery
10. Watercress, apple, cucumber, garlic
11. Asparagus, carrot and celery
12. Carrot, celery, parsley and cabbage, onion, sweet basil
13. Carrot, coconut milk and ginger
14. Carrot, broccoli, lemon, cayenne
15. Carrot, sprouts, kelp, rosemary
16. Apple, carrot, radish, ginger
17. Apple, pineapple and ginger
18. Apple, papaya and grapes
19. Papaya, cranberries and apple
20. Leafy greens, broccoli, apple
21. Grape, apple and blueberries
22. Watermelon (alone is best)

Enjoy Healthy Fiber for Super Health
From UC Berkeley Wellness Letter

- KEEP BEANS HANDY, probably the best fiber sources. Cook dried beans and freeze in portions. Use canned beans for faster meals.
- EAT BERRIES, surprisingly good sources of fiber.
- INSTEAD OF ICEBERG LETTUCE, choose organic green lettuces, romaine, bib, butter, etc., spinach or cabbage for variety salads.
- LOOK FOR "100% WHOLE WHEAT" or whole grain breads. A dark color isn't proof; check labels, compare fibers, grains, etc.
- WHOLE GRAIN CEREALS. Hot, also cold granola with sliced fruit.
- GO FOR BROWN RICE. It's better for you and so delicious.
- EAT THE SKINS of potatoes and other organic fruits and vegetables.
- LOOK FOR HEALTH CRACKERS with at least 2 g. of fiber per ounce.
- SERVE HUMMUS, made from chickpeas, instead of sour-cream dips.
- USE WHOLE WHEAT FLOUR for baking breads, muffins, pastries, pancakes, waffles and for variety try other whole grain flours.
- ADD OAT BRAN, WHEAT BRAN AND WHEAT GERM to baked goods, cookies, etc.; whole grain cereals, casseroles, loafs, etc.
- SNACK ON SUN-DRIED FRUIT, such as apricots, dates, prunes, raisins, etc., which are concentrated sources of nutrients and fiber.
- INSTEAD OF DRINKING JUICE, eat the fruit: orange, grapefruit, etc.; and vegetables: tomato, carrot, celery, broccoli, cabbage, etc.

Wherever flax seed becomes a regular food item among the people, there will be better health. – Mahatma Gandhi

---

Wherever you go, no matter what the weather, always bring your own sunshine. – Anthony J. D'Angelo

Fasting Cleanses, Renews and Rejuvenates

Our bodies have a natural self-cleansing system for maintaining a healthy body and our *river of life* – our blood. It's essential that we keep our entire bodily machinery healthy and in good working condition from head to toe!

Fasting is the best detoxifying method. It's also the most effective and safest way to increase elimination of waste buildups and enhance the body's miraculous self-healing and self-repairing process that keeps you healthy.

If you prepare for a fast by eating a cleansing diet for 1 to 2 days, this can greatly facilitate the cleansing process. Fresh variety salads, fresh vegetables and fruits and their juices, as well as green drinks (alfalfa, barley, chlorophyll, chlorella, spirulina, wheatgrass, etc.) stimulate waste elimination. Live, fresh foods and organic fruit and vegetable juices can literally pick up dead matter from your body and carry it away. Following this pre-cleansing diet you can start your liquid fast.

Daily, even on most days during our fasts, we take 3,000 mg. of mixed Vitamin C "Emergen-C" powder (C concentrate, Acerola, Rosehips and Bioflavonoids) in liquids. This is a potent antioxidant and flushes out deadly free radicals. It also promotes collagen production for new healthy tissues. *Vitamin C is especially important if you are detoxifying from prescription drugs, alcohol or stress overload,* stated our friend, famous scientist Dr. Linus Pauling.

A moderate, well-planned distilled water fast is our favorite or a diluted fresh juice (35% distilled water) fast can help cleanse your body of excess mucus, old fecal matter, trapped cellular, non-food wastes and can help remove inorganic mineral deposits and sludge from your pipes and joints. Fasting works by self-digestion. During a fast your body intuitively will decompose and burn only the substances and tissues that are damaged, diseased or unneeded, such as abscesses, tumors, excess fat deposits, excess water and congestive wastes. (See benefits page 154.)

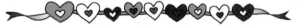

The nation badly needs to go on a healthy diet. It should do something drastic about excessive, unattractive, life-threatening fat. It should get rid of it in the quickest, safest possible way and this is by fasting. – Allan Cott, M.D.

Fasting is Your Body's Miracle

Even a short fast (1-3 days) your body will accelerate elimination from your liver, kidneys, lungs, bloodstream and skin. Sometimes you will experience dramatic changes (a cleansing and healing crisis) as accumulated wastes are expelled. With your first few fasts you may temporarily have headaches, fatigue, body odor, bad breath, coated tongue, mouth sores and even diarrhea as your body is cleaning house. Be patient with your body!

After a fast your body will begin to respond and healthfully rebalance. When you follow Bragg Healthy Lifestyle, your weekly 24 hour fast removes toxins on a regular basis, so they don't accumulate. Your energy levels will begin to rise – physically, psychologically and mentally. Your creativity will begin to expand. You will feel like a *different person* – which you are – as you are being cleansed, purified and reborn. Fasting is an exciting and wonderful detox cleansing and miracle healing blessing for your body.

Excerpt from **Bragg:**

(153)

Dr. Nikolayev, Director of a famous Russian Fasting Clinic, often quotes an old German proverb: **"The illness that can't be cured by fasting can't be cured by anything else."** *Fasting permits the miracle cleansing and healing powers of the body and the mind to assert itself to cleanse and heal.*

Dr. Nikolayev – who fasts several times a year in 7, 10 to 15 day stretches stated, "I usually fast for prophylactic reasons. I also fasted several times with a scientific purpose to make an experiment. I always feel excellent when I fast. It's always a happy, restful time."

Dr. Nikolayev discovered that his patients responded to fasting treatment after all other forms of therapy had failed. The patients had been chronically ill and felt hopeless about their future life! Most of them would have never functioned again. Fasting gave them a new fresh recharged lease on life.

Allan Cott, M.D. noted in his book – Fasting, The Ultimate Diet *that "75% of patients treated by fasting improved so remarkably that they were able to resume an active life!" –* (amazon.com)

The human body has one ability not possessed by any machine – the body has the ability to repair itself. – George W. Crile

The Bragg Healthy Lifestyle followed daily will help you enjoy a long, healthy life!

BENEFITS FROM THE JOYS OF FASTING

Fasting renews your faith in yourself, your strength and Gods strength.
Fasting is easier than any diet. • Fasting is the quickest way to lose weight.
Fasting is adaptable to a busy life. • Fasting gives the body a physiological rest.
Fasting is used successfully in the treatment of many physical illnesses.
Fasting can yield weight losses of up to 10 pounds or more in the first week.
Fasting lowers & normalizes cholesterol, homocysteine & blood pressure levels.
Fasting improves dietary habits. • Fasting increases pleasure eating healthy foods.
Fasting is a calming experience, often relieving tension and insomnia.
Fasting frequently induces feelings of euphoria, a natural high.
Fasting is a miracle rejuvenator, slowing the ageing process.
Fasting is a natural stimulant to rejuvenate the growth hormone levels.
Fasting is an energizer, not a debilitator. • Fasting aids the elimination process.
Fasting often results in a more vigorous marital relationship.
Fasting can eliminate smoking, drug and drinking addictions.
Fasting is a regulator, educating the body to consume food only as needed.
Fasting saves time spent marketing, preparing and eating.
Fasting rids the body of toxins, giving it an internal shower & cleansing.
Fasting does not deprive the body of essential nutrients.
Fasting can be used to uncover the sources of food allergies.
Fasting is used effectively in schizophrenia treatment & other mental illnesses.
Fasting under proper supervision can be tolerated easily up to four weeks.
Fasting does not accumulate appetite; hunger pangs disappear in 1-2 days.
Fasting is routine for most of the animal kingdom.
Fasting has been a common practice since the beginning of man's existence.
Fasting is a rite in all religions; the Bible alone has 74 references to fasting.
Fasting under proper conditions is absolutely safe. • Fasting is a blessing.

154

Fasting As A Way Of Life – Allan Cott, M.D. – find on Amazon.com
Fasting is not starving, it's nature's cure that God has given us. – Patricia Bragg

Spiritual Bible Reasons Why We Should Fast

Acts 13:2-3	Neh. 1:4	Luke 4:2-5, 14	Deut. 8:3-8	Matthew 9:9-15
Acts 14:23-25	Ezra 8:21	Luke 9:1-6, 11	Joel 2:12	Matthew 17:18-21
3 John 2	Gal. 5:16-26	Mark 2:16-20	Matthew 7:7-8	Deut. 11:7-14, 21
1 Cor 10:31	Gen. 6:3	Matthew 4:1-4	Psalms 119-18	Neh. 9:1, 20-21
1 Cor. 13:4-7	Isaiah 58:6, 8	Psalms 69:10	Psalms 35:13	Matthew 6:16-18

Dear Health Friend,

This gentle reminder explains the great benefits from *The Miracle of Fasting* that you will enjoy when starting on your weekly 24 hour Bragg Fasting Program for Super Health! It's a precious time of body-mind-soul cleansing and renewal.

On fast days I drink 8-10 glasses of distilled (our favorite) or purified water, (I add 1-2 tsps Bragg Organic Vinegar to 3 of them). If just starting, you may also try herbal teas or try diluted fresh juices with $^1/3$ distilled water. Every day, even some fast days, add 1 Tbsp of psyllium husk powder to liquids once daily. It's an extra cleanser and helps normalize weight, cholesterol and blood pressure and helps promote healthy elimination. Fasting is the oldest, most effective healing method known to man. Fasting offers great, miraculous blessings from Mother Nature and our Creator. It begins the self-cleansing of the inner-body workings so we can promote our own self-healing.

My father and I wrote the book *The Miracle of Fasting* to share with you the health miracles it can perform in your life. It's all so worthwhile to do and it's an important part of The Bragg Healthy Lifestyle.

With Love, *Patricia*

Paul Bragg's work on fasting and water is one of the great contributions to The Healing Wisdom and The Natural Health Movement in the world today.
– Gabriel Cousens, M.D., Author of *Conscious Eating & Spiritual Nutrition*

Chapter 15

Doctor Rest

Sound Sleep is Necessary To Build a Strong Heart

Primitive men and women arise at daybreak and the early hours of their days are spent in vigorous physical activity. About mid-day they eat their largest meal and then immediately afterward they lie down to rest or take a nap (just as babies, young children and even animals do). In an hour they wake up refreshed – ready for the 2nd half of the day. They are active again until sundown, and shortly afterwards go to sleep again. So primitive man is awake about 12 hours and sleeps about 12 hours.

Modern, civilized man drives himself all day under high-pressure. His day is filled with stresses, strains, worries and cares. A daily nap or *siesta* is unknown to the routine of most people. All day long he takes many stimulants to keep himself going – coffee, tea, alcohol, pills, cigarettes, excessive amounts of sugar, candy, chocolate, ice-cream, etc. – everything to try to keep his poor body up to the constant *go, go – push mode*!

He lives in this hectic, fast driven age and at night he has brilliant lights and action to keep him awake. His amusements and entertainments all begin at night. The night clubs turn on bright lights and loud music. Movie theaters lure him into films that are promoting sex, crime and violence. TV, web, videos, radio, parties – everything seems to be geared to stimulate him. Instead of going to bed for much needed sleep he drives himself, chasing happiness and peace of mind.

When he gets sleepy he just takes a pill, and to keep him awake, drinks some strong coffee, then to relax he has some poisonous alcohol. He is constantly straining his nervous system – all of which has a disastrous deadly effect on his circulatory system and his heart.

Think of yourself as a "battery" – you discharge energy and you must recharge yourself with proper food, sleep and constructive emotions.

The majority of American's nerves are so frazzled and burned-out that it's often impossible for them to get a good night's sleep. As a result, *they consume sleeping pills and tranquilizers* to calm their exhausted nervous systems. It's no wonder that, in addition to the *soaring heart disease rate in the United States*, we have more people with mental disorders than ever before in history. A half-million American men and women are committed to mental institutions every year. These facilities are now so over-crowded that they represent one of our society's greatest medical and financial problems today. For peaceful, calm and healthy nerves read the Bragg book *Build Powerful Nerve Force*. See back pages for book info.

Sleep is Essential To Life Itself

You cannot have a strong heart, a sound mind and a healthy nervous system if you do not get enough good and sound restful sleep! Sleep is essential to building and maintaining a strong, vital heart. *Sleep is more necessary than food!* Anyone can fast on water for days – or even weeks if necessary – without any serious harm if they are well-nourished before beginning the fast and have a satisfactory food-supply after its conclusion. But no one can *fast* from sleep for a few days without side effects. Man can't endure an entire week of sleeplessness.

In early English history condemned criminals were put to death by depriving them of sleep. This forced sleeplessness, in fact, has been used as a form of torture and execution by the Chinese and is more feared than corporal punishment. Those subjected to this always died raving maniacs! Sad facts illustrate the necessity of sleep!

Take a Daily "Siesta"

If you want to build a *strong heart* and *nervous system*, take a mid-day nap. Getting hour's rest in middle of day is like having 2 days in 1, because when you wake up after your mid-day nap or *siesta* you have stored up a terrific nervous energy reserve. We believe the people of Mexico, South America, Spain, France and Italy had a healthy idea when they followed the long established policy of closing down businesses from noon to 2 pm. for lunch and siesta. Rest is important for building a powerful body and heart!

How Much Sleep Do We Need?

How much sleep do we need? Every individual is different. Some people require more sleep than others. Those possessing the greatest vitality and the strongest constitutions require less sleep than those of limited vitality and weaker recuperative powers. Those who possess a strong metabolic system and great vitality can store energy during sleep and they also recover from the exertions of the preceding day more rapidly. A strong person will be restored more quickly than others. Their system can more rapidly repair the wear and tear of their daily work than that of a weaker individual.

Newest University of Chicago research has found strong signs of *accelerated* ageing in healthy young men after less than a week in which they slept for just four hours per night. Not getting enough sleep can age people prematurely and promote illness! Getting 12 hours of sleep for several nights turned the students back to their right age.

Most people need 7 to 8 hours of sleep nightly. Women and children require 9 to 10 hours sleep. We feel that 8 hours of sleep per night is important for a strong heart and that 1 to 2 hours of this sleep should be obtained before midnight. A single hour of sleep before midnight is worth 3 hours of sleep after midnight. We enjoy short half hour afternoon naps when possible – the siesta habit is great!

157

Rules for Restful, Recharging Sleep

It's best to *sleep with your head to the north*, so you will be in direct contact with the Earth's vibrations, and on an outside porch or in a room with good cross-ventilation. Weather permitting you can sleep nude or in non-constricting natural (cotton, silk, wool) garments. Sleep with a head cradle pillow so that your neck and spine are aligned and your heart won't have to pump so hard against gravity. Sleeping in a cramped position, on a soft mattress (firm is best) or in a manner that blocks circulation is not conducive to restful sleep. In bed, stretch and spread your body out, then practice slow deep breathing and sleep peacefully.

A study at College of Holy Cross in Massachusetts found students who got less sleep, got poorer grades! Teens need 8 to 10 hours sleep per night.

Your Mattress is Your Best Sleeping Friend

You should sleep on a firm mattress or place a board under a soft one. This allows the muscles to stretch in natural relaxation and relieves pressure on vital organs.

When on our world lecture tours, we often have to move our mattresses onto the floor to be firmer. It seems that some of the world's top hotels put their money into showy lobbies and not into firm mattresses. We also often find old, sagging mattresses in many of the homes we visit – but new cars in their garages! At our Desert home we had new wood platforms made. A firm mattress goes on top of this board with four legs on castors. Try a miracle foam mattress pad on top of the mattress – it's great. It might take you a few nights to become accustomed to being stretched out flat – but soon your body will thank you with more energy.

We travel all over the world in trains, planes, ships, buses and automobiles and often use soft foam ear plugs to shut out unnecessary sounds and noises. We feel it's absolutely necessary that we sleep in a place that is quiet! Even though we often do fall asleep when there is noise all about us, the vibratory action of the noise can have a direct effect on the heart, circulation and nervous system.

We believe that individuals should sleep alone. Two people sleeping in one bed is not healthy because there are always toxins being released from the body and these toxins can be absorbed. Then there is also the noise of a person who breathes too deeply, snores (page 160), or is restless – all of which interferes with the other person's sleep. It has been proven by scientific research that a person gets a better night's rest and stores up more vitality when they sleep alone. Married couples will wake up more refreshed sleeping next to each other – each in their own twin bed. If this is not acceptable, then a king size bed is certainly preferable to the usual small double bed.

Research shows that sleep deprivation increases the risk of high blood pressure and heart disease. Sleep deprivation can change the body's secretion of hormones. These changes promote over-eating and alter the body's response to sugar intake – changes that can promote weight gain and increase the risk of developing diabetes. – Newsweek Magazine

America's National "Sleep Debt"

A National Sleep Foundation poll back in 1998 discovered that a whopping 67% of American adults have a sleeping problem and that over one-third, (37%) are so sleepy during the daytime that their daily activities are interfered with. Over the past 100 years, we've reduced our average sleep time by 20% and, over the last 25 years, added an additional month to our annual work-commute time. Thus, our national *sleep debt* is rising and while our society has changed, our physical bodies and needs have not. We are paying a dear price for progress!

Getting Enough Sleep Lately?

The odds are you aren't getting sufficient sleep. American adults presently average 7 hours nightly. While everyone's sleep needs vary, scientific research indicates that we require at least 8 hours of sleep nightly.

Few are lucky enough to enjoy 5 to 6 hours of sound sleep and still perform well at work; to just get caught up, a full ten hours of rest is frequently called for!

159

Before Calling it a Night . . .

First make a conscious choice about how you wish to spend the 30 to 45 minutes before bedtime. Avoid a rush to *get things ready for tomorrow* or to catch up on tasks not completed during the day. Slow down your body and mind with an aroma-therapeutic/massage bath and enjoy a soothing lemon balm tea drink before bedtime and a melatonin (1mg.) cap aids sleep, plus fights free radicals.

Try Lemon Balm for a Night So Calm

Lemon Balm, whose scientific name is *melissa officinalis,* is a cooling plant with both nervine and antiseptic qualities. As a member of the Labiatae family, which also includes peppermint and spearmint, lemon balm is native to most areas of Europe and has been widely grown worldwide. Flowering between June and October, its lemon-like fragrance is unmistakable.

Help me to know the magic of rest, relaxation and the restoring power of sleep.

Like restful camomile, it's lemon balm's primary, volatile oils that make the plant medicinal. While appearing to be just a simple plant, it delivers a wide range of rather potent cures, ranging from stomach pain to the worst cases of insomnia. Try lemon balm tea before bedtime – miraculous results have been reported and it can be blended with a variety of herbal teas. Also others to try for sound sleep are: Sleepytime, skullcap, valerian herbal teas, magnesium and calcium supplement and melatonin (1 mg) before bedtime.

Tips for Healthful Sound Sleep

- Avoid stimulants such as caffeine, found in coffee, tea, chocolate, soda, and nicotine, found in cigarettes and other tobacco products.
- Don't drink alcohol to "help" you sleep.
- Exercise regularly, but be finished with your workout routine no sooner than 3 hours prior to bedtime.
- Establish a regular and relaxing bedtime routine; for example, try aromatherapy bath or shower.
- Associate your bed with relaxing, recharging sleep – don't use it for doing work or watching TV.
- If you often suffer from insomnia, don't take naps.

Relief for the Snorer in the House

Now there are choices in treatment for relieving snoring. The first breakthrough is a simple nasal strip (adhesive band-aid-like device) that helps keep open nose's nasal passages and allows easier airflow during sleep. Available at pharmacies, sizes small to large.

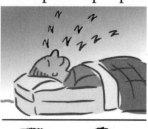

The second is RIPSNORE™. A simple, one-piece device that molds to the shape of your mouth. The device is very flexible when being fitted. It stops snoring or drastically reduces snoring in 98% of people who started using it. The RIPSNORE™ holds the lower jaw slightly forward,

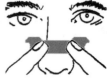

moving base of tongue away from back of airway and soft palate - allowing throat to be opened and the snore to be silenced. The device is almost identical to dental ones, but is a lot more affordable. To order on web: *ripsnore.com*

Safer, Non-Invasive Tests & Natural Therapy

Heart Surgery Versus Natural Therapy

Unfortunately, our Western medical professionals too often turn first to invasive procedures rather than safer and less expensive non-invasive, healthier alternatives. This is true in both diagnosis and treatment.

An *angiogram* is an invasive and dangerous diagnostic test (causes approximately 20,000 deaths yearly) that is supposed to measure blood flow and blockages in the heart. A catheter is inserted into a patient's leg artery (through the groin), and threaded up through the artery all the way to the patient's heart. A National Heart, Lung & Blood Institute study found this painful invasive procedure is a shocking 82% inaccurate! Nevertheless, doctors continue to prescribe expensive angiograms. In the years since the study, angiograms performed in the U.S. have risen from 380,000 to well over one million yearly!

Expensive treatment for heart disease is increasingly dominated by invasive procedures. In the 17 years between 1979 and 1997, coronary bypass surgeries increased a shocking 432% – from 115,000 operations to 607,000 performed yearly! If only this trend reflected a growing, positive effectiveness of these invasive procedures – but this is not the case! These and current studies prove it!

A recent Harvard University medical study reports that invasive heart surgeries have little effect on the long-term survival of most heart patients. Only in the most severe cases did dangerous, invasive operations show significant statistical merit. The study suggested that these types of surgeries could be reduced by 25% or more without endangering the health of heart patients. Rather than using this important study's advice, doctors are increasing expensive heart surgeries at an alarming rate!

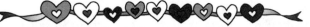

Harvard School Public Health Study found 84% of those who sought a second opinion after scheduling heart bypass surgery, were told they didn't need it!

Safer Minimally Invasive Surgery

Recent advances have now brought the open heart surgery technique to a viable safer alternative. Minimally Invasive Surgery was originally conceived by a Russian Surgeon in the early 1960's. The procedures are now performed through an incision less than $1/3$ the size of a drastic full sternotomy (the former ranges from 9-12 cm long, the latter averages 30 cm). Two types of procedures are being done using this technique: minimally invasive direct coronary artery bypass, or MIDCAB, and minimally invasive valve repair and replacement. MIDCAB is the "beating heart" surgery since the heart doesn't have to be stopped or placed on cardiopulmonary bypass (the heart-lung machine that oxygenates the blood and maintains blood pressure) and surgeons can operate while the heart continues to beat, which is safer for the patient. Due to the reduced incision size, this newer technique is less traumatic, has shorter recovery time that helps reduce the need for pain-killers. For more information visit web: *www.heartsurgeons.com*

The Safer Road to Reduce Heart Disease

Dr. Julian Whitaker, one of America's famous heart specialists, became so outraged years ago over unsafe trends that he says, *"I gave up being a surgeon to become a healer."* He founded the renowned Whitaker Wellness Institute in Newport Beach, California, and has the nation's leading health newsletter, *Health and Healing*. A healthy lifestyle like The Bragg's Lifestyle is his alternative to angiograms and surgery. *(drwhitaker.com)*

Dr. Dean Ornish, the Clinical Professor of Medicine, School of Medicine, UC San Francisco, is another world famous doctor-turned-healer. When Ornish's heart patients embraced a healthy, energetic exercise regime and ate only nutritious, low-fat foods, their heart conditions began improving within one month! After a year, most patients had virtually no chest pains or heart problems! For 82% of his patients a healthy lifestyle reversed their arterial clogging! *(www.pmri.org)*

Many patients who undergo heart bypass surgery suffer significant and long-lasting loss of brain power. It is better to follow Dr. Dean Ornish, other wise doctors and the Bragg Healthy Lifestyle – who advocate a 100% healthy lifestyle.

Non-Invasive Tests for the Heart

The safer, less expensive, non-invasive alternatives can bring about greater health. The invasive heart tests and operations are extremely dangerous, expensive and often unnecessary! There's a growing number of doctors that specialize in protecting heart patients from the use of angiograms, bypass surgery and angioplasty. As an alternative to invasive testing procedures, they place sonar devices, electronic sensors, microphones, etc. on the outside of the chest. These sensitive tests can usually judge heart disease better than procedures which use dangerous, invasive catheters, tubes and needles.

When needed, consult with some of the health physicians and organizations that are dedicated to make the healthcare of your heart a wise, safer job. Here are some sources:

- 💜 **Life Extension**, Ft. Lauderdale, FL • For Health Advisors 1-800-226-2370 • *www.LifeExtension.com*

- 💜 **Dr. Dean Ornish**, PMRI Institute, CA • For Heart Retreats (800) 775-7674 x221 • *www.pmri.org* or *my.webmd.com*

- 💜 **The Whitaker Wellness Institute**, Newport Beach, CA 1-800-488-1500 • *www.whitakerwellness.com*

- 💜 ACAM (American College for Advancement in Medicine) (888) 439-6891 for telephone assistance & Physician Link.

For list of U.S. holistic doctors see web: *www.acam.org*

We tend to think of advances in medicine as being a new drug, a new surgical technique, a new laser, something high-tech and expensive. We often have a hard time believing that the simple choices that we make each day in our diet and lifestyle can make such a powerful difference in the quality and quantity of our lives, but they most often do. My program consists of four main components: exercise, nutrition, stress management, love and intimacy – these promote not only living longer, but living better. – Dean Ornish, M.D.

It's better to be safe than sorry. Medical and Hospital Emergency Centers do fast tests to relieve your mind to see if you have had a mild heart attack.

SURVIVING A HEART ATTACK WHEN ALONE

Since many people are alone when they suffer a heart attack, this is very important for without help, the person whose heart stops beating properly could lose consciousness in seconds. Taking deep breaths and coughing deeply repeatedly every 2 seconds until the heart beats normally again and until help comes could save your life! The deep breaths get oxygen into the lungs and coughing movements squeeze the heart, to help keep blood circulating and that will help it regain normal rhythm. – www.mendedhearts.org

Tests Reveal Risks of Heart Disease

It is often said that you're probably not at risk for heart disease if your LDL (Low Density Lipoprotein) level is low (see inside front cover). However, a recent study published in the American Heart Journal concluded that almost half of the patients with cardiovascular disease actually had low LDL levels (less than 100mg/dl). This is contrary to standard belief! According to the National Cholesterol Education Program, new risk factors for heart disease include high amounts of small, dense LDL. This type of LDL is dangerous, it can be easily oxidized by free radicals (see page 26) and can penetrate into the delicate inner lining of the blood vessel walls to form plaque. In contrast, large LDL do not put you at increased risk. This may sound confusing, but by taking these special tests, you may be able to detect heart disease more efficiently.

• **LDL Test:** A special test done to measure the type of LDL you have (large or small), and another LDL test that measures lipoproteins (see inside front cover).

164

• **High-sensitivity C-Reactive Protein (CRP) Test:** CRP is an independent risk factor for heart disease, a known inflammatory compound that could be damaging to the blood vessel walls, setting you up for plaque formation, inflammation and possible heart attack (see page 44).

• **Homocysteine Test:** Homocysteine is a by-product of your body's metabolism. When high it can increase inflammation of your blood vessel walls (see page 45).

• **Fibrinogen Test:** Fibrinogen is a blood clotting factor, if it is high, you are at risk of forming blood clots that could lead to a heart attack or stroke. Braggzyme Systemic Enzyme supplement helps maintain a more normal inflammatory response and helps maintain safe fibrin levels for a more healthy cardiovascular system.* See page 212 & 256.

These specialized tests can give a much better picture of your risk for heart disease. But even if your results from all these tests are within normal ranges, you will still be wise when you choose to follow the Bragg Healthy Lifestyle.

Read Natural Choices for Women's Health *by Dr. Laurie Steelsmith available on* www.amazon.com *and* www.DrSteelsmith.com

MRI – Non-Invasive Window into the Heart

Doctors use *magnetic resonance imaging* (MRI) as a non-invasive, diagnostic tool to look at soft tissue inside patients without having to invade the body. MRIs use a powerful, but harmless magnetic field that reveals in great detail, shape and condition of your internal organs. Doctors use this test to diagnose various heart and entire body conditions.

What can non-invasive MRI procedure tell a doctor about patient's heart and circulatory system? *Miracle* MRIs identify heart scarring and any other indications of previous or future heart attack. It can reveal arterial clogging and presence of any foreign masses in and around heart and body. It detects signs of heart disease, identifies vascular disorders (enlarged heart, etc.) and checks vessel health. Warning: MRIs cannot be used on people with pacemakers or arterial clips.

Beware of 3-D Image Heart Test

According to study (*cnn.com*) in *New England Journal of Medicine*, an expensive CT scan that uses multiple x-rays to produce 3-D heart images can't replace the more traditional coronary Angiography for finding blocked blood vessels in patients with chest pain.

"I think it's (x-rays with 3-D images) being used without clear data of any benefit for the patient," says Dr. Rita Redberg, a Professor at University of California, San Francisco School of Medicine. "The usefulness of CT scan is debatable and the test has risks! The scan exposes patients to more radiation than an angiogram. These patients may need an angiogram anyway, as well as other tests that could expose them to even more radiation, like those that use nuclear tracers. We don't know what the radiation risks are, it's been estimated that we're going to see tens of thousands of additional cancers because of our increased use of CT scans!" Dr. Redberg adds, "It's not always true that more tests are better and it drives up our health-care costs without clear benefit to the patients."

Resveratrol, quercetin, green tea extracts (non-caffeine), soy products, genistein, polyphenols, BBI enzyme (from soybeans), antioxidant nutrients, herbs, spices & plant extracts can offer substantial protection against risks of radiation-induced cancer in X-rays & CT scans. As many as 29,000 cancers are caused each year from CT & other radiology scans.– LifeExtension.com

Seek These Safer and Healthier Non-Invasive Tests for Heart Disease:

DOPPLER COLOR FLOW IMAGING TEST This is a safe, non-invasive imaging ultrasound. It shows a clear profile that checks the entire blood vessel system simultaneously. When needed, doctors check for possible blood slow-down and blockages that can cause future heart attacks and strokes, and even death. See web: *www.aarogya.com*

ELECTROCARDIOGRAM & CARDIOKYMOGRAPHY It's an **EKG** and **CKG** graph that records heart electrical activity. The heart has an electric current running through it. The heart contracts and pumps blood throughout your body. This contraction is started off by an electric current, even though it is a weak one. This current begins in a part of the heart called the sino-atrial node, or the pacemaker, which sets the pace for the heart to beat. From the pacemaker this current follows a well-defined path through the rest of the heart. This movement can be recorded by electrodes, which are plastic plates placed on the chest and limbs to detect current flow inside heart. The graph recorded is the **EKG and CKG, both painless tests.** These tests detect disturbances in the beating pattern of electrical activity in the heart, called arrhythmia. They also check if any chamber of the heart is abnormally enlarged or if any of the walls have thickened. (See web: *www.AmericanHeart.org*)

166

ECHOCARDIOGRAPHY This painless ultrasound is an examination of the heart, used to evaluate structural conditions like the thickness of the walls; the way the heart walls move during exercise or rest; diagnose valve trouble; inflammation; congenital heart disease and congestive heart failure. Echocardiography uses high-frequency sound waves to produce images of the heart. A small transducer, like a microphone, passes over the chest, sending out impulses that bounce off the heart. The transducer records these echoes, and a computer converts them into a graphic display on the screen.

Doctors may now be able to detect "silent" heart disease when CKG test is used with electrocardiograms (EKGs). A recent study revealed that EKGs alone missed 39% of heart disease cases. When the CKG test was added to EKGs, then only 8% of cases went undetected.

EXERCISE STRESS TESTING This is an exercise EKG electrocardiogram that's performed with controlled exercise such as a treadmill. The patient's maximum heart rate is calculated based on their sex and age, then the patient is connected to the EKG machine and exercises until the heart is beating steadily at the calculated rate. This test shows changes in the EKG pattern, especially for those with narrowing of the coronary arteries. If blood pressure drops during the test, this could be another sign of coronary artery disease. The stress test is also used for people who recently recovered from a heart attack, as an initial step in assessing the heart's blood supply. Please express any sensations experienced during testing (sometimes it's too much too soon). This test can detect coronary artery disease in 75% of cases.

NUCLEAR SCANNING This safe technique uses radioactive materials known as isotopes, to examine the heart. The isotopes used are harmless substances, and are less radioactive than most x-rays. In nuclear scanning, the patient is given a small dose, either orally or injected. These isotopes flow through the blood system giving off radiation which is photographed by a special camera producing pictures of the heart. These pictures show how well the ventricles are working and where there is scarring, damaged or oxygen-starved areas of the heart.

HOLTER MONITOR is a portable version of an EKG. It records heart rhythm (pulse) during your daily activities. Worn for 24 hours or more. The heart waves are picked up by electrodes or patches placed on chest. Waves are recorded on tape inside the monitor. This recording is then scanned into a computer for analysis. Holter Monitors are used on patients who experience chest pain, dizziness, palpitations or fainting, which is often caused by narrowing of arteries or heartbeat abnormalities. It may also show evidence of silent ischemia, like an angina attack (page 17) without chest pain. (web: *www.heartsite.com*)

FDA ALERT: CT Scans are causing widespread radiation overdoses!
Machines have no "red light" that says they are over-radiating. Hospitals are intentionally using high levels of radiation to get clearer images. Overdose symptoms include: headaches, memory & hair loss, rashes, seizures, stroke symptoms & confusion. Patients have higher risk of brain damage & cancer. Reducing mistakes is important, but it's better to eliminate unnecessary tests!

New Millennium Health Technology Provides Safer, Faster, Better Testing

DIGITAL TECHNOLOGY can take a routine test like a chest x-ray to a new height of quality and has many advantages. It's an environment saver because there are no film processing chemicals utilized; it is safer for the patient since it uses lower x-ray doses and reduces need for retakes and more exposure; it gives an instant picture and can be stored on a computer and transmitted instantaneously to the doctor's office, the hospital or anywhere required! (See web: *www.MayoClinic.com*)

PET SCANNER: **Positron Emission Tomography** is a unique 32-ring scanner that can detect and measure metabolic activity throughout the body and especially the brain. It pinpoints the source of cancers, neurological and heart diseases; thereby reducing all the expensive, unneeded operations, exploratory surgery and hospital stays! The PET scanner saves time, money and most important, precious lives! (See web: *www.radiologyinfo.org*)

FOR SURGERY: XKNIFE STEREOTACTIC RADIOSURGERY uses a radionic *invisible blade,* not a scalpel; this makes surgery non-invasive, bloodless, and reduces complications, discomfort, and hastens recovery. Excellent for brain tumors and arteriovenous malformations (AVMs). (See web: *www.radionics.com*)

Dr. Paul Dudley White of Boston – Famous Heart Specialist's Wise Words

Dr. White, the former president of the American Heart Association, world famous pioneer heart specialist and our friend, gave this wise advice on taking care of the heart. We want to call your attention especially to the following points made by Dr. White in an article written for the American Heart Association. He begins with his startling facts that *middle age begins at 20,* and the *dangerous years are ages 20 to 40!* Here's Dr. White's words.

The only thing that is truly yours that no one can take away from you is your attitude. So if you take care of that, everything else in life becomes much easier.

Dr. White, when does middle age begin? "At age 20, and it lasts until 80. And the dangerous years of this span are the first 20 years, not the last. These are the years when an overfed and under-exercised public is sowing the seeds of a coronary harvest. I conceive the ages of man as five. Birth to the 20th year; then a three stage middle age of 20 to 40, 40 to 60, 60 to 80; and finally old age – 80 to 100. The latter constitutes a steadily expanding horizon to which I see no eventual limit. Our life expectancy should keep rising indefinitely as research keeps making progress against disease." (Genesis 6:3)

Unlimited Life Expectancy is Possible!

Dr. White stated, "The public can play an important role in this effort to push the life-span farther and farther. Physical-fitness and nutritional programs for men and women between the ages of 24 and 40 would guard against creeping degeneration and would instill lifelong good health habits."

"A man marries sometime in his 20s; his wife cooks too much and too well – and between her cooking, the family car, the web, video games and the TV, the man has gained maybe 20 to 40 pounds by the time he's 45. These are the years in which atherosclerosis (cholesterol blocking and clogging the arteries) and rusting of the arteries occur. This can ultimately reach the brain as a stroke, or the heart as a coronary thrombosis (massive blood clot). It may also affect the kidneys. This is why an apparently healthy man drops dead at 45 or 50. His death is not sudden at all; an unhealthy lifestyle has silently been building up for years!"

"The automobile and the TV, I might add, should be the servants of the American public, not its masters. Despite the nation's generally unhealthy way of life, two factors work in favor of the American person, Dr. White concludes. It is never too late – at any age – to begin controlling obesity and resuming a program of sensible exercise and a healthy diet. One excellent form, available to all, is walking. This should be brisk, and for a normally healthy person five miles weekly is not enough. Neither is one weekly 18-hole golf game.

Those who love deeply never grow old; they may die of old age, but they die young.
– Benjamin Franklin, printer, inventor – bifocal glasses, started library. (1706-1790)

There you have it – from Dr. White, known as Dean of American Cardiology. Exercise and diet can be regular and enjoyable parts of the Healthy Lifestyle as you will discover by following this Bragg Heart Fitness Program we are outlining for you. *(www.heartprotect.com)*

Dr. Carrel's Successful Eternal Life Study

Dr. Alexis Carrel, eminent biologist and Nobel Laureate, of the Rockefeller Institute in New York City, *proved* to the world that *living flesh can be deathless!* In 1912, this Nobel Scientist took a sliver of a heart muscle from a chicken embryo and provided it with 2 essentials of life – simple protein food and correct drainage for the tissues. His simple laboratory experiment kept this tiny piece of embryo heart flesh tissues alive for 35 years.

This 35 year study proved that the heart tissue could have continued indefinitely! In 1912, Dr. Carrell received the Nobel Prize for this cell biology work. At the end of the experiment in 1947, this heart tissue had lived many average chicken lifetimes – the equivalent of hundreds of years of human life! It was called the *tissue of eternal youth.*

This amazing bit of embryo heart flesh doubled its size every 48 hours! Slices had to be cut away and discarded daily because its continued growth would have made it impossible to feed and cleanse the living heart cells. At the Rockefeller Institute, any scientist could observe eternal life before their very eyes! We can learn an important lesson from Dr. Carrel's revealing scientific demonstration with the tissues from a chicken heart. Namely, that if the body is correctly fed and its poisons and wastes are properly eliminated, life can continue indefinitely! (See Dr. Carrel on web: *www.nobelprize.org*)

170

What you eat and drink or whatever you do
– do it all to the glory of God and your human temple – your body.
– 1 Corinthians 10:31 and 3 John 2 are Bragg Crusades mottos

It's magnificent to live long if one keeps
healthy, alert, youthful and active. – Harry Fosdick

Positive affirmations create miracles. – Beatrex Quntanna

Quietness and Cheerfulness is important and to give thanks at meals is most essential for health and happiness. – Oliver Wendell Homes

---

A laugh is just like sunshine, it freshens all the day. – Heart Warmers

Paul C. Bragg & Mentor – Bernarr Macfadden

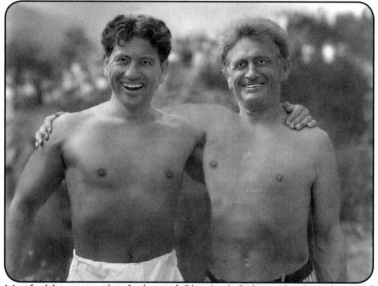

Macfadden was the father of Physical Culture in America and Bragg the father of the Health Movement and the originator of Health Food Stores. Paul C. Bragg began his life-time career in Natural Physical Fitness at the turn of the century by working with the famous Physical Culture pioneer, Bernarr Macfadden. Bragg was editor of Macfadden's Physical Culture Magazine, the first publication to bring the basic principles of healthful living to popular attention in the U.S.A. They were credited with "getting women out of bloomers into shorts, and men into bathing trunks." Bragg started Macfadden's "Penny Kitchen Restaurants" during the big Depression Era, when they fed millions of hungry people for a penny each. Bragg helped develop America's first Health Spa at Dansville, New York, where this photo was taken. Bragg then opened Macfadden's Deauville Hotel, which gave undeveloped Miami Beach, Florida its great new beginning.

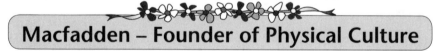

Macfadden – Founder of Physical Culture

My dad was associated with Bernarr Macfadden, who spent thousands of dollars to find the *oldest living humans* on earth. Dad was his main researcher on this project. This took my dad to many interesting, remote parts of the world, interviewing men and women from *103 to 154 years of age!* Dad found this work fascinating, because in his heart he always wanted to live a long life; not just the life of the average person which ends at about 74-78, but an active life that would last 120 to 150 years. His research proved it can be done! Now many scientists worldwide are agreeing.

Zora Agha – Age 154 – Secret of Youth – Healthy Foods and Hard Work (Exercise)

In Constantinople, Turkey, my father met and talked with an amazing man named Zora Agha, who was 154 years old. What was this remarkable man doing at age 154? He was a baggage porter for the large railroad station. For 12 hours every day he carried heavy baggage! His eyesight, hearing and physical strength were unbelievable! His mind was keen and he had a sense of humor that kept him joking and smiling all day long.

Through an interpreter, my dad questioned Zora Agha about the secrets of his astounding, long and healthy life. *His whole diet was simple* and uncomplicated. It included no refined or processed foods. Never in his life had he eaten refined white bread or sugar and – being a Moslem – he had never tasted any alcoholic drinks.

Dates Are Longevity Enhancers

When asked what his favorite food was, Zora replied readily, *dates* (see web: *www.DatesAreGreat.com*). The reputation of dates as a longevity enhancer has been verified by other research on long-lived, healthy people. We discovered that people who eat dates have more vital energy, stamina and endurance. At one time, in the Atlas Mountains of North Africa, Dad was investigating a tribe of primitive Arabs who astonished him with their energy and extraordinary strength. He met men 70, 80 and 90 years old who were expert horsemen and could spend days in the African heat of 120°–130°F without cause to worry.

But it was from Zora Agha in far-off Turkey that we first learned of the amazing value of dates as a healthful food. Dad also learned that he limited himself to 3 or 4 dates at a time. Zora knew the remarkable energy value of the *natural sugars found in dates*, but he also knew the body has only a limited capacity for handling these sugars, and so did his teeth. In 154 years of life he lost only 2 teeth! Dad was amazed when he displayed his teeth and gums. Every tooth in his mouth looked like a pearl – perfect, strong, white and hard. All Americans would be envious.

Periodontal disease increases the chance of a heart attack. See pages 193 & 223

Zora's Longevity Diet is the Biblical Diet

The vigorous 154 year-old Zora Agha also ate large amounts of garlic, one of humanity's *forgotten foods*. Garlic has been called *the poor man's penicillin* and as Nutritionists, we know its value in helping to keep the heart and arteries fit. (More on garlic and the heart later.) Zora also said he ate only stale *black bread that had been dried in the sunshine*. He would purchase a loaf of black bread, slice it and let it dry in the sun. He never ate fresh bread. (Note: When traveling, we dry our health bread in the sun by putting it on the window sill. See, you can even have healthy, sun-dried bread when traveling.)

Other items of Zora's humble diet included ripe olives and lots of organic sun-dried dates, fruits and vegetables, greens and only occasionally lean meat and some eggs. He didn't use butter. The only oil he used for salads and cooking was olive oil. This healthy, natural oil has been used in Europe, Turkey, throughout Asia Minor and in the Holy Land, for hundreds of years. Zora's only beverage besides *water* was *mint tea*, which is the traditional beverage of all Arabs and Moslems. It occurred to my father that Zora Agha had naturally discovered the secrets of longevity. This was also the secret of the old Biblical Patriarchs who lived to fabulous ages and whose diet was so much like Zora Agha.

Life's Quantity and Quality Depends Upon the Food We Eat and Our Activity

From this 154 year-old, healthy, energetic man we learned a great deal about keeping the heart fit by means of a simple natural foods diet and vigorous exercise.

Dad met only one Zora Agha in his lifetime. But we know that when the mass of civilized, humankind adopts a simple natural diet with exercise and keeping active, then there will be more people who will reach Zora's remarkable age.

With exercise you can become young at heart, literally, improving the heart muscle's ability to adapt quickly and help reduce the risk of heart attack & stroke.

Now learn what and how a temperate diet will bring great benefits along with it. In the first place, you will enjoy good health. – Horace 65 B.C.

When you have been stricken by illness, your new car, your new home, your new big, bank balance – all these fade into unimportance until you have regained your vigor and zest for living again. – Peter J. Steincrohn, M.D.

Every intelligent person will agree that life's length and quality depends largely upon the food we eat. How carefully we select our foods will logically depend on how sound our heart, brain, nerves, body cells, tissues and vital organs will be tomorrow, next month, next year and 10 years from now. *The chemistry of the food a person eats becomes the chemistry of their body.*

Face the Challenge – Change Your Bad Habits

Face this challenge and start changing your bad habits of living into good, healthy habits. This is both a mental and a physical process. Your mind must control your body! Never let the body be in command! That is the duty of the mind. It must command the body to absolute obedience to its will. The whole person is at its best when mind and body work as a team. Then you can enjoy more Supreme Health!

Health, Happiness and Longevity – It's All Up to You!

174

The results back up our teachings. You, and only you, can take proper care of your heart and body so that you may enjoy the *prime of your life* indefinitely! Most people reach their *prime* between 25 and 35, and then experience a decline. People who follow this Bragg Heart Program can attain the prime of life at any age and maintain and enjoy it for life! Now, plan and follow it!

If you have high or low blood pressure, you can restore it to normal by following the natural laws that keep your heart in good condition. My father's blood pressure always averaged 120 systolic over 70 diastolic, with a pulse rate in the 60s – just like a young man! We know that his case is not an isolated one – he's not a freak of perfect health. In our years of health consulting we have met countless men and women in almost unbelievably good physical condition at high calendar ages.

Researchers have discovered the more healthy habits an individual practices, the longer they live and the healthier they are! – Elizabeth Vierck, *Health Smart*

Our habits, good or bad, are something we should & can control. – Dr. E. J. Stieglitz

Nine men in ten are suicides caused by their living habits. – Ben Franklin

Chapter 17

A Frank Talk Concerning Cardiovascular Disease

Build Yourself a Healthy Heart

We believe in prevention. We agree thoroughly with the American Heart Association when it says that the heart needs daily exercise and a healthy, balanced diet with ample fruits and vegetables in order to remain healthy.

We believe that the first thing you should do is to live life so that you will not damage your heart. General public knowledge of the heart is crammed with fallacies as well as facts. Let's consider some of these misconceptions that we so frequently hear about:

Should the Heart Patient Always Rest?

No! The belief that a *coronary* always means the end of an active life is widespread – and quite wrong! Most coronary occlusions (heart attacks) involve only a small branch of the *coronary tree* or system of blood vessels. The blocked artery may be naturally bypassed by the collateral channels which lie unused in the heart tissues awaiting just this eventuality. The new circulatory route may be so efficient that the patient may have no disability at all after recovery! Remember – ***Your Body is a Miracle.***

Certainly the process of healing is assisted if the body is rested during recovery. The degree and duration of any activities should be decided by your doctor. Once healing is complete, too much rest rarely achieves anything of value. To the contrary, it is likely to increase disability by adding ill effects of physical unfitness and loss of self-confidence.

Remove physiological stress from the body, and the body does what it was designed to do, it heals itself! – Dr. Ben Johnson, founder of "The Healing Codes." Featured in the movie The Secret • www.thehealingcodes.com

What lies behind us and what lies before us are small matters compared to what lies within us. – Ralph Waldo Emerson

Faith can place a candle in the darkest night.

Is Exertion Harmful After a Heart Attack?

This is a variation of the same theme as the need for rest and is usually just as wrong. The heart has enormous reserves of power which are seldom – if ever – used in ordinary living. It is this reserve which enables individuals to perform apparently superhuman feats in times of crisis or in an emergency. Athletes constantly call upon this reserve – the runner who covers a mile in 4 minutes, for example, or the 50-mile endurance swimmer.

The reserve power of the heart is not greatly decreased and is available for use even after many heart attacks. It should not be abused, of course. Generally, the heart patient who over-exerts himself will develop warning symptoms – some chest pain, angina and maybe even some breathlessness. This is Mother Nature's Way of telling him to slow down. Similar symptoms, however, may be the result of physical unfitness, unusual stress or some tension, or emotional upsets and fatigue.

The thing we want you to remember is that *your body is always undergoing change*! You are not now the same person that you were a minute ago. The body is always undergoing endless change, for better or worse. Every moment of your life old cells are being sloughed off and new, healthy ones hopefully are taking their place!

The question you must ask yourself is, *What kind of new cells am I making for my body? Am I building these new tissues with healthy food or unhealthy food?*

If you drink alcohol, coffee, tea, cola drinks and eat refined white bread, refined sugar, salted or rich, fatty foods you are going to make weak body cells that will prematurely decay, causing you health problems! On the other hand, if you follow the instructions given in our Healthy Heart Fitness Program, you are going to help build a stronger heart and a stronger body. It's all in your hands! We can only guide you to help yourself!

If you have had a heart condition, start today to systematically and efficiently build a fit heart and strong circulatory system. Please don't think *a bad heart* means a permanent farewell to those healthy activities which are a major part of the enjoyment of life – it isn't!

According to studies done in the book, *8 Steps to a Healthy Heart* by Robert Kowalski, life after heart problems can be rich and fulfilling, but only if the patient and his family take the steps needed to assure that recovery includes treatment of both mind and body. Attending a cardiac rehabilitation program is beneficial for both the patient and family members, there they can share their feelings with other patients who have gone through cardiac experiences. It bridges families together and gives support to those in need. Mended Hearts, Inc. is highly recommended and offers help, support, and encouragement to heart disease patients and their families. Ask your hospital for your local Mended Hearts chapter or write them at: **Mended Hearts, Inc.,** 7272 Greenville Avenue, Dallas, TX 75231. Or call them at 1-888-432-7899 (See web: *www.mendedhearts.org*)

Our Opinion of Heart Transplants

We do not personally believe in heart transplants. When the first heart transplants were announced the newspapers reported every detail. The average person wants to hear this kind of news. They always want the easy way out. If your heart goes bad, just have another put in! Sounds wonderful! Why take care of your heart when you can get a new one when the old one falls apart? The first experiments with heart transplants were, of course, done with animals. The medical researchers reasoned that if heart transplants would work on animals, they would work on humans. Dr. Barnard of Africa performed heart transplants on 50 dogs and they all died.

Heart Transplants – Risky and Costly

If success were judged during the first 24 hours after the operation, it would have been rated a success. After 2 days, complications arose, the same rejection problems that could not be solved in the animal experiments. (Interesting: pigs and human hearts are similar in size, etc.)

The body survives in a hostile environment only because it can fight off the invasion by toxic poisons, bacteria, viruses and other foreign matter. The same mechanism attacks the transplanted heart and can slowly destroy it. This difficulty was apparent also in early kidney transplants, with a survival rate of 5% (today it's 95%, but requires daily use of costly toxic drugs with side effects). The major problem in heart and kidney transplants is tissue rejection. The body wants nothing to do with a foreign object – and that's exactly how it views the new organ! No matter how healthy the new heart or kidney may be, it's not a natural part of the body it's being placed into (example: wood splinter in finger). To date medical science has found nothing natural – only immuno-suppressant drugs – which helps to overcome this rejection of new tissues or organs by the body, and in our opinion, they never will.

According to American Heart Association the average wait for a new heart is between 6 months to three years, which jeopardizes the waiting patient's health and results in high astronomical medical bills! A heart transplant operation will cost over $148,000 and to maintain it, will cost over $20,000 per year for life! Take care of your precious heart – start living The Bragg Healthy Lifestyle!

Risk Factors Angioplasty & Stent on Women

Heart attack is the leading cause of death in women annually. Women who undergo angioplasty are twice as likely to die than men are, stated researchers at the Montefiore Medical Center and Albert Einstein College of Medicine in New York. "This study is significant because we compared men and women for the same procedure, angioplasty, and for the same condition, heart attack. We found women to have 2.5 times the risk of dying during their hospitalization compared to men," said top cardiologist Dr. David L. Brown. The researchers looked at 1,044 patients, they found that women undergoing stent and angioplasty for a heart attack are more severely ill and had more diabetes, obesity and hypertension than did the men.

Pacemakers Save Lives When Needed

Famous Dr. Earl Bakken pioneered 1954 the first transistorized pacemaker. Medtronic, company he co-founded, has developed a new pacemaker for ailing hearts that has and is saving thousands of lives. Dr. Bakken lives in Hawaii and is a big Bragg Liquid Aminos fan. (earlbakken.com)

Chapter 18

The Art of Longevity

The best recipe for a long life is to keep living The Bragg Healthy Lifestyle. There is no substitute for this!

Consider each day a little life in itself – make it as perfect and well-rounded as you can! Try to have a stronger heart and better health on your next birthday than you have today. By living supremely for the moment you are living superbly for a long, healthy, happy future!

You must always be self-aware of your life! The moment you relax your guard the enemy is ready to rush in and smite you in your heart. True, with luck, you may live long without trying, but you will live longer and better if you exert an effort. Living for longevity is an art. The person who deliberately sets out to prolong their days has a healthy chance of doing just that!

Forgetfulness of self may make the time go like magic, but it does not help build a strong heart and keep you youthful. Inattention to yourself and the carelessness that results is extremely dangerous! As you live longer you should grow less objective and more subjective. The more self-centered you are, the better you will conserve your precious health resources. Longevity often belongs not to those who forget themselves for others, but to those who are most health conscious of themselves and their physical, mental, spiritual and emotional well-being.

This may seem to give the long-lived a positive, strong, at times selfish character. Not at all! Without healthy nourishment we cannot aspire to fulfill our dreams. To seek to prolong one's life is to extend one's term of usefulness and service. We aren't advocating you prolong your life at the expense of others! Rather, we suggest that you live a long, healthy life so that you may be more useful to your family and others, as well as to yourself!

It's important for people to know what you stand for. It's equally important that they know what you won't stand for! – Mary Waldrip

A man is as old as his arteries – his river of life. – Virchow

179

Secret of Longevity – Organized Resistance

The secret of longevity is to understand that *the enemy is not your chronological age. Premature ageing is preventable!* You must put up a strong defense against ageing. There are a few, of course, who are born with such wonderful constitutions `they simply can't kill themselves. You might find a few octogenarians who say they owe their long life to smoking, alcohol and avoiding exercise. You can tell them confidently that they could extend their lifespan by a good 20 years by living a healthy lifestyle.

Scientific longevity is organized resistance. It is based on a knowledge of the body and the laws of health. Above all, it means reliance on Mother Nature. She abhors ill health, which is another name for toxic poisoning and clogged pipes. She is always striving to purify and to vitalize. She wants to help you if you will only let her. Medicine, drugs and doctors will do you no good if Mother Nature is not backing them up.

Heart Disease is Your Greatest Threat

Remember that you must always defend yourself against coronary thrombosis (heart attack), stroke, hypertension (high blood pressure), arteriosclerosis (hardening of arteries), atherosclerosis (blockage and clogging of the arteries by cholesterol and other debris), angina pectoris, varicose veins and other cardiovascular (heart and blood vessel) diseases. *Diseases of the heart and circulatory system are the #1 Killer in the United States* taking more than a million American lives each year – more than all other causes combined! And never forget that you must also guard against stiffening joints, fibrous tissues, deafness, blindness and many other enemies of health and life.

All this means that there must be a little slowing of activity. We believe the advice *grow old gracefully* is wrong! Mother Nature and God will eventually decree the end – but until then it's far better to live life as youthfully as possible! You are *as old as you feel – so feel young!* When you abide by Mother Nature's Laws, you feel younger! By trusting in and obeying Her laws, understanding your miracle physical machine and how to care for it, you can live a longer, more youthful, healthy, happy life.

Old Age is Not Inevitable – Scientists Say Man Should Live to 140 to 185

It seems to us that what we call *old age* is the result of sluggish cell action in the body. The cells are being renewed all the time by the moisture in the lymph circulation, just as a tree is renewed all the time by the circulation of its sap. But if the cell is clogged in any way by toxic deposits which it cannot be completely rid of – chiefly because of poor circulation of the blood – it cannot then make full use of the building material brought by the lymphatic system or the new health nourishment and oxygen delivered by the bloodstream.

On the basis of what we have done with rabbits, we have come to the conclusion that if we can do the same thing for man, he can live a healthy and normal life until the age 185! A waxy material, cholesterol, is deposited on the arteries and there is a correlation between age and the amount of cholesterol deposited. In tests of 52 rabbits, we have been able to reverse the symptoms of old age! says a brilliant Brooklyn Polytechnic Institute Biochemistry Professor, Dr. W. M. Malisoff, who did extensive research there.

Biologists tell us that man grows an entirely new body every 11 months. That being the case, why does mankind age? Scientists answer this by saying that the body fails to shed all of the old cells. As we stated earlier, deposits in the cell prevent its full use of the new material. So instead of living 7 times the period it takes man to mature, as most animals do, man's life is unnaturally shortened by his unhealthy lifestyle. Sad facts!

Confirmation of this statement comes from Dr. Serge Veronoff of Paris, France, who says that each of us should live to be 140 years old. A human being matures at 20 years of age. Mother Nature constructed the human machine to live 7 times that age, or 140 years. The fact that some men and women even today have been able to reach or surpass the age of 120 years and have then died of some disease seems to prove the validity of the 140 year life-span without disease as natural.

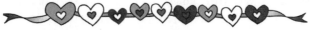

Man's days shall be to 120 years. – Genesis 6:3

#1 Cause of Death – Coronary Disease

Deposits in the arteries retard the circulation of the blood. The speed and efficiency of the bloodstream has a great effect upon the prolongation of life. It is the bloodstream which provides the entire body with the required nourishment and oxygen before it removes harmful substances for elimination. Slowing of blood circulation, loss of elasticity of blood vessels and disturbances of the machinery which regulate distribution of blood are among the most important causes of the shortening of life, vigor and health.

In our opinion, there is no physiological principle limiting health or human lifespan. We believe that radiant health and youthfulness is within reach, but it must be earned. This is your life! It is your sacred duty to yourself, Mother Nature and God to learn now and how to keep your body healthy and fit for a long lifetime!

The #1 cause of widows and widowers in the United States is coronary (heart) disease. Remember our discourse of cholesterol, and the fact that high cholesterol levels are invitations to heart attacks? Statistics show that cholesterol levels in American men, and now women also, increase rapidly between ages 30 and 65. Be on guard! Cholesterol should be tested by all twice a year.

Women before the age of 50 used to be much better protected against degenerative artery disease than men. Today women have achieved an unfortunate equality by developing heart attacks and strokes with more frequency than men. Statistics show 53% of women die of heart disease compared to 42% of men. The scientific theory that female sex hormones play an important part in providing protection against the harmful menace of atherosclerosis is apparently true – but not powerful enough to offset the deadly effects of an unhealthy lifestyle! (See risks and symptoms for women pages 38-39). As soon as menopause starts in women, the protection of these sex hormones ceases, they claim, and they become just as susceptible as men to heart attacks and strokes. It's important, women of all ages should not neglect their heart health. (I've never taken hormones – only natural supplements and occasionally use wild yam cream. – PB)

Unhealthy Lifestyle Living is Slow Suicide

Just because you are *feeling fine* does not mean that you can afford the risk of continuing to choke your bloodstream with the high cholesterol diet typical of most people in our *modern* civilization. Bacon and eggs, meat, potatoes, pies and cakes, bread with butter or margarine, milk and ice cream, all the rich foods that most men and women crave are slow poisons to your heart and circulatory system. Remember that these poisons work silently and insidiously. Their effect may not become evident until you suddenly have a heart attack. Always remember the wise words of famous Dr. Paul D. White:

"Death from a heart attack is not sudden, it had been building up for years by your lifestyle and eating habits!"

Your Family's Life is in Your Hands

We would like to suggest to everyone that you re-read Dr. White's warning and that you take it seriously. If you want to keep your family alive, work on them to exercise every day as you watch what you feed them and yourself! You may be shortening the lives of your family with too many fattening and highly saturated foods. Their lives are in your hands! You prepare and put the food on the table for your family to eat. You will learn from this valuable book how to keep your family in perfect health! Follow these instructions and soon you and your family will discover a startling increase in vigor and vitality, with a sense of well-being.

Remember that young people can also die of heart disease! Teach your children how to eat correctly. Give your family more fresh salads, more lightly steamed vegetables, more fresh fruit desserts. Eliminate gravy (it's loaded with cholesterol). Eliminate dairy products. Enjoy healthier soy, rice and nut milks. Serve delicious herbal teas such as mint, alfalfa, chamomile, lemon balm and banish coffee and the salt shaker from your table! Your reward will be a radiantly happy, healthy family. Use Bragg's *Vegetarian Recipe Book,* it has over 700 recipes and hundreds of healthy ways to feed yourself and family! (See back pages for book list.)

Enjoy Lighter, Smaller Vegetarian Dinners

It seems to be an American custom for people to eat their biggest meal in the evening. From a standpoint of heart attacks, this is the worst time to eat a big meal . . . especially a meal with a preponderance of fat. It has been definitively established by researchers that the blood is more likely to clot 2 to 8 hours following a meal with a high fat intake. It would therefore seem logical to avoid heavy meals – particularly in the evening – to minimize the chances of intravascular clotting. The occurrence of a heart attack after eating a heavy meal has been recognized by doctors for years. Just think how often you read or hear about a man in his prime dying of a heart attack during his sleep at night or in the morning.

Retired people, of course, can regulate their meal-times easily. Business people can dine at an earlier hour in the evening and can certainly regulate their diet to promote their health and prolong their lives.

184

A light healthy vegetarian meal is ideal for evenings.

It can begin with a raw combination salad with lemon and olive oil dressing. Follow it with 2 lightly cooked vegetables such as green beans, zucchini, peas, corn on the cob, kale, okra, vegetable chop suey, etc. Several nights a week add a baked potato – but do not drench this potato in fat! Season it with Bragg Sprinkle (24 herbs & spices) or Bragg Kelp and a spray of Bragg Aminos and Bragg Organic Olive Oil instead of butter.

Now we are not telling you that the price you must pay to avoid a heart attack and live a longer life is to give up good flavor. Not at all! As mentioned previously, delicious French dishes, soups, salads, potatoes, veggies, etc. are world famous and among the best heart-healthy recipes. A good French chef rarely uses salt and cooks with very little fat. The secrets of French flavor are in the use of herbs, garlic, olive oil, onions, green peppers and mushrooms.

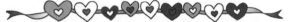

I've seen sickness and asthma disappear completely in response to major shifts in diet and lifestyles, as eliminating sugar, milk, meat and switching to healthier, vegetarian diet. – Dr. Andrew Weil, www.drweilselfhealing.com

Prevention is always preferable to the cure!

Chinese Recipes Promote Heart Health – America's Coronary Disease Rate is Ten Times Higher than China!

The Chinese have a low cholesterol, low fat diet – in sharp contrast to the high cholesterol, high fat diet found in the United States, Canada and the more prosperous countries of Europe. Pathologists, scientists and medical researchers have produced overwhelming evidence that when blood cholesterol and fats are high, the arteries suffer from a greater degree of atherosclerosis. **Atherosclerosis has always been a "disease of the rich"**. Only those who could afford rich, fatty foods have been heart attack and stroke victims. The heart and blood vessel degenerative diseases have historically been associated with royalty and wealth. Cholesterol was found in the mummies arteries of the Pharaohs of Egypt, whose diet was far richer than their subjects.

Today we have millions of people in our Western industrialized countries who can easily afford rich foods. You hear and read about *the affluent society and its blessings.* But this affluence is exacting a high price in atherosclerosis and the nearly epidemic number of heart attacks, strokes and cancers now happening worldwide.

Millions of people living in China and other Asian countries are rarely afflicted with heart disease. Their main dietary item is, and has been for centuries, one of the most healthful of all vegetables: the soybean. Soybeans contain a high percentage of unsaturated fatty acids and lecithin, two good preventives of heart disease.

The basic Chinese diet consists of rice and lightly cooked vegetables, with meat used only as an occasional flavoring. When you order chicken or beef chop suey in a Chinese restaurant, you always get a plentiful dish of vegetables such as celery, onions, green bellpeppers, bamboo shoots, water chestnuts and soy and bean sprouts – flavored by only small amount of thinly sliced chicken or beef and a bowl of rice (ask for brown rice). No bread and butter is served at an authentic Chinese Restaurant.

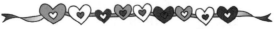

You are what you eat, drink, breathe, think, say and do. – Patricia Bragg, ND, PhD.

Our Favorite Chinese Recipes
Raw Combination Garden Salad

Slice cabbage into bite-size pieces. Add sliced carrots, celery (greener the better), turnips, radishes, cucumbers, tomatoes, fresh chopped parsley and spinach. Toss with a dressing of Bragg Liquid Aminos, Bragg Organic Olive Oil and Bragg Organic Apple Cider Vinegar or fresh lemon juice, or try delicious Bragg Ginger & Sesame Dressing.

Mushroom Chop Suey

With a sharp knife slice onions, green bellpeppers, celery, chard or kale, carrots, bok choy, cabbage and any other vegetables you desire. Mix with fresh or canned bean sprouts, water chestnuts, bamboo shoots. Try a variety of fresh mushrooms. Put these mixed vegetables into hot wok or skillet with small amount of unsaturated oil as olive, corn, soy or safflower oil. Add sliced garlic if you enjoy it. (We do. We feel that garlic purifies the body's pipes and helps boost immune system.) Stir in Bragg Sprinkle (24 herbs & spices), Bragg Kelp, 1 tsp. of Bragg Aminos or spray it over chop suey. Add Bragg Nutritional Yeast before serving, adds a delicious seasoning flavor.

The secret of Chinese food is not to overcook it! Sauté this chop suey mixture 8 to 12 minutes at the very most, stirring constantly with a wooden spoon.

Healthy Organic Brown Rice

Brown rice is a healthy staple food. Use organic brown rice – 1 cup of rice to 3 cups distilled water. Add 1 teaspoon Bragg Liquid Aminos and 1 teaspoon Bragg Organic (extra virgin) Olive Oil. Cook in double boiler or thick-bottomed pan with tight lid, over medium heat until soft and fluffy (20 to 30 minutes). Don't stir until ready to serve, then add another dash or spray of Bragg Liquid Aminos, Bragg Sprinkle, Bragg Kelp, Bragg Organic Olive Oil and Bragg Nutritional Yeast Seasoning for delicious flavors. Serves 3 to 4.

Fresh Fruit Dessert

A fresh organic apple, pear, banana or any other fresh fruit in season will top off this perfect heart-smart meal.

You Can Teach Old Dogs New Tricks

They say you *can't teach an old dog new tricks*. We feel wise, mature humans have the intelligence to protect themselves from heart attacks by learning new tricks of eating. It's worth the effort to know that you are not going to wake up one night gasping for air and clutching your heart! Start now improving your daily lifestyle habits!

To avoid heart attacks you must learn to substitute Bragg Organic Olive Oil instead of butter, margarine and other clogging, saturated and hydrogenated fats. If you are a milk drinker, learn to substitute the rice, almond or soy milks and drink these instead of cow's milk. Learn to use herbs, kelp, garlic, onions, Bragg Liquid Aminos, and Bragg Sprinkle (24 herbs & spices) and Bragg Kelp Seasoning to add delicious flavors and aromas instead of salting your foods. Also, you know the saturated fats in meats, and dairy products are your enemies! Learn to eat them sparingly or best not at all! *Keep meals as natural and simple as possible.*

Most people shake their heads in doubt when they are told they must give up using salt. It does take a little time to make the change from salt to naturally delicious and nourishing herbs, kelp and Bragg Aminos. We told you that the salt craving is acquired and not natural. It will disappear, just as Dad's cravings did. You will find that your 260 taste buds will soon reject salted foods.

Feel Youthful Regardless of Your Years

Life is the survival of the fittest and no one – yes, no one – is going to be able to protect your heart except you! It's your duty and responsibility to yourself to live a healthy lifestyle so that your heart can remain strong and healthy throughout your entire natural lifespan.

We must live by knowledge and wisdom – not by old wives' tales and myths. That is why this book was written: to provide the scientific facts about your heart and outline a Heart Fitness Program that helps you take care of this marvelous, life-giving machine.

Becoming more aerobically active with daily active exercise in middle or old age now has a lot more bearing on your current heart health, than having been sedentary in your 20's to 40's. It's what you do today that counts, get busy, eat healthy and start brisk walking today!

This book's message is simple. It tells what a heart attack is, what causes it and what you can do today to prevent it. We offer no magic formula or cure for heart trouble. In this Heart Fitness Program we have simply brought together well-documented evidence from the great scientific and medical researchers, statisticians and dietitians of the world. The medical world is relying upon heart transplants, surgeries and drugs. We are not the least interested in heart transplants nor in the diagnosis and treatment of heart troubles. We are mainly interested in disease prevention by keeping the heart healthy and fit! Let's stop heart troubles before they start! Why wait for the heart to deteriorate before we do something about it? We must live healthy today, so that we don't have a heart attack tomorrow! What we sow in one period of our lives, we reap in another. Let's sow seeds of good health so that we will automatically have a powerful, fit heart.

You can definitely capture and retain the joyous feeling of youthfulness no matter what your calendar years may be! By living The Bragg Healthy Lifestyle outlined in this Heart Fitness Program, you can again regain the joy of youthfulness and boundless energy.

Don't let people drag you down to their low level of thinking. *You are as young as your arteries!* Decide that you are going to live a healthful life to help keep your arteries and heart years younger. Keep your *thinking* youthful and you will feel young again! Age is not birthdays – it's a matter of how well you live, feel and enjoy each day of your life!

It's Never too Late to Think Youthfully

This whole Heart Fitness Program is designed to make you forget birthdays and live a more youthful, carefree life. Living by this philosophy of life prevents many physical and mental miseries that are likely to afflict older people. In this way you can maintain health, strength, vigor and happiness as the years roll by. It has been said that *There is really no cure for old age – only those who die young escape it.* But our Heart Fitness Program can really help you feel and look younger and enjoy living longer.

Cardiovascular disease is not the inevitable result of ageing.
Healthy preventive measures can be taken to avoid heart disease.
– James F. Balch, M.D., Co-Author "Prescription for Nutritional Healing"

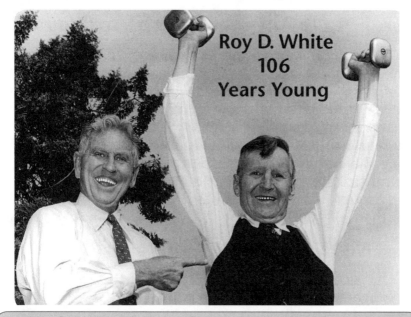

Roy D. White
106
Years Young

Paul C. Bragg with His Youthful Friend

Here's Roy White on his 106th birthday – yes, you read correctly – 106 years young! Roy D. White lives in Long Beach, CA. He had a keen brain, a great sense of humor and a feeling of youthfulness tingling throughout his supple and active body. Roy can lift both hands high overhead, keep his knees stiff and bend over and touch his toes – an exercise people half his age can't do. And he never fails to walk his 5 miles a day. Being a widower, Roy takes care of his own apartment and prepares his own meals. At 106, he appears to be a youthful, active 75 years young and even with the physical agility of a man many years younger.

Remember that throughout this Heart Fitness Program we have stressed how important it is to keep physically active. Our claims are backed up by this 106 year old youngster! Don't let your circulation slow down!

To over-rest is to rust and rust can lead to destruction.

Roy believes his daily brisk walks help him physically, mentally, emotionally and spiritually. He believes you can walk off your tensions and worries. Roy says, *I've always been free from tensions – that's the foundation of my Philosophy of Life. Fear and hatred are the two worst things in the world. You can multiply your troubles by thinking they're worse than they are – no matter how mean anyone has been to me, I've never hated them. Let them do the hating, not me!*

Forgiving & Forgetting Keeps You Youthful

Tensions, anger, greed and excessive emotionalism can damage your heart! Roy is an example of the great philosophy of forgiving and forgetting! He says most young children think that way and he wants to always be kind and think youthful. When you have a strong sense of well-being and optimism, your entire attitude toward life is fresher and more youthful! Your whole philosophy can change to a younger and more optimistic one, replacing the stagnating defeatist attitude many people have. When you feel youthful, you act youthful and then all your actions and thinking are more youthful!

We No Longer Celebrate Birthdays

That is absolutely right. No more birthdays for us! We no longer want to measure our lives by calendar years – only by healthy, biological years. Yes, we both have lived wonderful long lives. Dad to a great-great-grandfather. But this does not stop us from enjoying our youthful activities. We're going to continue to play tennis with the youngsters, climb the mountains with the mountain climbers, swim with the swimmers and dance with our young health friends – and the seniors who are still young at heart! One of Dad's favorite dancing partners is a girl of only 88 – but what a dancer! She is as graceful as any of his great-granddaughters!

Don't think the years are making you old – it's the way you live that preserves or damages your heart and arteries. You must earn your bonus years! You must earn your youthful arteries! You must work hard to preserve the vitality and the fitness of your heart and your body! It's wonderful when you buildup a fit heart and body, for then you find more time and energy for so many more activities than you did when you were stumbling around tired and only half-alive. When you have a heart that is beating joyfully, the world looks like the Garden of Eden. You become a carefree person with a song in your heart, a sparkle in your eye and a spring in your step. Life can be beautiful – for when you're healthy, you're happy! After all, is that not the greatest goal in life – *sweet, contented happiness and inner peace!*

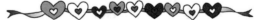

Each birthday is the beginning of your own personal fresh new year! Your first birthday was a beginning, and each birthday is a chance to begin again, to start over, to take a new grip on life. – Paul C. Bragg, ND, PhD. Life Extension Specialist

Chapter 19

Chelation Therapy

Miraculous Method of Unclogging the Arteries

We want to share with you a miracle of medical science which we found so amazing that we researched it thoroughly. We have found mounting impressive clinical medical evidence, by our personal investigation, demonstrating a safe and reliable therapeutic method to counteract the terrible ravages of arteriosclerosis and atherosclerosis. These degenerative diseases arise from hardening and clogging of the arteries.

This method is Chelation (pronounced key-lay-shun) Therapy. It has been proven effective to the point of being termed *miraculous* by physicians as well as patients. *It's totally incredible!* declared John, the first chelation therapy patient we interviewed. We met John through a mutual friend from Chicago, who was visiting us at our desert home in California. He insisted that we go to John's home in nearby Palm Desert to learn firsthand of his friends *miracle cure* and it was a miracle for sure!

A leading heart specialist had told John, a man in his 40's, that he had a life expectancy of maybe 2 years unless he underwent drastic surgery for a *3-way bypass;* i.e., transplanting blood vessels from his leg into his heart to bridge or *by-pass* blockages in 3 arteries (with 100%, 95% and 75% blockages respectfully). Even if he survived the surgery, there was no guarantee that similar blockages would not reoccur, leaving John in despair.

Through friends he learned about Ray Evers, M.D., who for many years had been achieving remarkable recoveries in similar cases with chelation therapy. The normal treatment period is 3 to 8 weeks and can be handled on an out-patient treatment at any of the doctors' offices or clinics that perform chelation therapy world-wide.

We met John 3 months after he had an 8 week series of chelation treatments under Dr. Evers' care. He had just had a checkup at famous Loma Linda Hospital and the tests showed no heart problems whatsoever!

Reversal of the "Ageing Process"

Shortly thereafter, we visited with Dr. Ray Evers at his Meadowbrook Hospital in Belle Chasse, Louisiana. He told us that over a period of 8 years he had treated over 10,000 patients with chelation therapy. Dr. Evers said that he believed *Chelation therapy could hold the key to the basic treatment of some of mankind's greatest killer diseases, all characterized by the same basic abnormality – that is, narrowing and closing off of the blood vessels, which can affect the health of every organ of the body.*

Everyone is familiar with the clinical picture of coronary or heart attacks, strokes or brain clots and hemorrhages, he continued, *but many other diseases such as diabetes, thyroid and adrenal disturbances, digestive problems, Alzheimer's, senility, emphysema, arthritis, multiple sclerosis, etc., may be caused in part, by interference with the proper delivery of blood, oxygen and nutrition to the vital cells.*

Chelation therapy attacks this basic problem of the cardiovascular system, Dr. Evers pointed out. *The results often produce significant relief of symptoms, are often life-saving and miraculous with patients being rejuvenated!*

192

We saw proof of his words with our own eyes. We observed people in their 40's to their 80's being brought into the hospital in wheelchairs – the victims of heart attacks and other circulatory or degenerative diseases such as stroke, diabetic gangrene, crippling arthritis and senility. Several weeks later we watched these same people walking out of the hospital with a new, reborn spring in their step, aglow with the joy of living!

What Causes This Amazing Rejuvenation?

The arteries of these people were being unclogged by chelation therapy, cleansed of the accumulated debris that had hardened and thickened the walls of their vital blood vessels. Now that their *pipes* were opened wide, the blood could once more course through their arteries, veins and capillaries to bring life-giving oxygen and nourishment to every cell in their body and carry off toxic wastes. The process of degeneration . . . commonly called the *ageing process*, was naturally being reversed!

What Mainly Causes "Ageing?"

As we discussed earlier in this book, the so-called *ageing process* is not the result of the passage of time, it is primarily the result of inadequate blood circulation, which can and does occur at any calendar age. *The chief villains are an excess of inorganic minerals, calcium, etc. and toxic chemicals (of which undistilled drinking water is a primary source), combined with an excess of cholesterol from a diet rich in saturated animal fats, hydrogenated fats and living an unhealthy lifestyle. All adds to the ageing process.*

Arteriosclerosis, or hardening of the arteries, can result from calcium deposits on the arterial walls. With the onset of deadly atherosclerosis, the calcified walls are further thickened by waxy deposits of cholesterol, which then dangerously narrow the blood passageway.

This abnormal calcium acts as a cementing agent and forms plaques with other inorganic minerals, and cholesterol and other waxy fats. This narrowing of the passageway, lessens both the quantity and force of the blood flow. Body cells degenerate from lack of nourishment and slowly drown in their own toxins, causing cells to die!

193

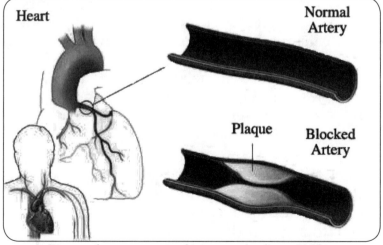

Diagram from: *www.naturalanswer.com/cardiocare101.htm*

Studies show low CoQ10 levels cause periodontal conditions, heart disease, declining memory and brain function. CoQ10 helped reverse these conditions.
– Dr. Stephen T. Sinatra, author, *CoQ10 Phenomenon,* and
The Sinatra Solution, Metabolic Cardiology • www.drsinatra.com

Chelation – Safe, Effective & Inexpensive Treatment For Coronary Heart Disease

Chelation therapy is a therapeutic adaptation of a natural biochemical process. The term *chelation* derives from the Greek word *chele* (pronounced keely) meaning a crab-like, pulling claw. Without going into detailed chemistry, chelation in human metabolism is the process by which an enzyme grabs or *binds* an organic mineral or *metal* and transports it to the body part where it can be utilized or removed. Example: Zinc to the pancreas for making insulin; and iron for the hemoglobin (red blood cells); calcium for building bones and its many other body uses; etc. (Remember, this refers to organic minerals – not inorganic, which cannot be used.)

This natural chelation process was not discovered until the 1940s. Its first therapeutic application was during World War II after a synthetic chelating agent was created to act as an antidote for *mustard gas* and other forms of arsenic poisoning. (For 20 years thereafter, chelation (pulling) agents were developed almost exclusively for ridding the body of toxic heavy metals such as lead.)

In late 1950 they discovered chelating agents used as poison antidotes were also effective in removing inorganic calcium deposits from the body's joints, organs and cardiovascular system. Through studies and medical research, a safe, effective chelating agent, known as EDTA by Abbott, was produced for removing these inorganic calcium clogging deposits and cholesterol plaques from the arteries and flushing them out the kidneys.

EDTA, a natural amino acid chelating agent, does not affect the normal organic calcium utilized by the body, but chelates only pathological inorganic calcium deposits. Chelation has proven an effective way to reverse hardening of the arteries. It unclogs the arteries by chelating out these atherosclerotic plaques, which then dissolve and break up. The cholesterol and other deposits then become slushy and are easily flushed out. All the residue *goes down the drain* and then the *pipes* of your cardiovascular system become more free flowing.

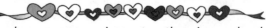

We must always change, renew, rejuvenate; otherwise, we harden. – Goethe

Chelation Therapy Includes a Healthy Diet

Carlos P. Lamar, M.D., of Florida, pioneered chelation therapy since 1960 and developed the basic procedures which have been so successful to date. These include the proper dosage of Endrate (ETDA) – delivered slowly intravenously, lasting from 3 to 4 hours per treatment.

As an essential part of chelation treatment, Dr. Lamar and his colleagues prescribe an anti-atherogenic diet that naturally chelates. Patients eat more frequent, lighter meals (with more tropical fruits; bananas, kiwis, mangos, papayas and pineapples, rich in the enzyme bromelain that acts like cardiovascular pipe cleaners) and eliminate dairy foods and saturated fats. Emphasis is placed on fresh, organic fruits and vegetables and natural foods.

Also, he gives them 50 to 100 mg. of vitamin B6 (pyridoxine) that controls sodium/potassium blood levels, that helps produce red blood cells and hemoglobin and protects against infection, plus additional vitamin and mineral supplements for each patient as needed.

Safe Diagnosis with Non-Invasive Tests

All patients are given thorough physicals and tests before the start of chelation therapy, and are carefully monitored during the chelation treatments, and given complete instruction for follow-up procedures. We were impressed with the infrared thermographic scan, which is diagnostic equipment that provides a safe, accurate method of locating and determining the degree of arterial blockage. Formerly this was done only by the dangerous angiogram test. This scan is a heat-sensitive instrument which records body temperature with direct correlation to blood circulation. This thermogram reveals location and degree of blockage by a light spectrum with a 10-color range. We don't recommended taking the risk of an angiogram. We endorse the non-invasive tests and the infrared thermographic scan on pages 163 to 168.

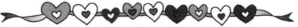

It's good that modern technology is available if you need it, but it's even better to prevent your arteries from getting plugged up in the first place.

Bragg Books can be your faithful health guides by your side night and day.

Chelation Therapy Promotes Natural Healing

Because it attacks the basic cardiovascular problem of degeneration, chelation therapy helps regenerate the body's natural self-healing and repairing powers. Natural blood circulation then restores normal metabolism and biochemical functions. The whole body *comes alive.* This is why chelation therapy, from the very beginning, has exceeded the wildest expectations of medical science.

When the first cases were reported back in 1964 by Dr. Lamar in the national medical publication *Angiology* (Vol. 15, No. 9, Sept. 1964), the most surprising result was the significant decrease in the insulin requirement of diabetics in response to chelation therapy. Two of the early cases were *hopeless* elderly diabetics with extreme mental deterioration and severe cardiovascular complications. After treatment there was a complete remission of symptoms, both physical and mental – plus a marked decrease in their insulin requirement. This *bonus* was attributed to the increased circulation in the pancreas, which promoted insulin production.

196

Since then, chelation therapy has been found to achieve such *bonus benefits* as regeneration and re-hardening of bones weakened by osteoporosis, restoration of mobility to frozen osteoarthritic joints, relief from hypothyroidism, reversal of prostatic calcinosis, recovery of normal functions of the kidney, other glands and organs and improvement in deteriorated retinas. There was improvement in all pathological conditions resulting from impaired circulation!

Chelation (ETDA) treatment has proven to be effective in treating heart disease. It also has achieved marked improvement in patients suffering from 2 of the most baffling central nervous system diseases – Multiple Sclerosis and Parkinson's disease. Perhaps the most spectacular results of chelation therapy are evidenced by the restored mental acuity in advanced senility cases.

In a landmark study, Dr. Carlos Lamar stated in the *Journal of American Geriatric Society* (Vol. XIV, No. 3, 1966), *"The physical rehabilitation and enjoyment of living experienced by these patients would be impossible to match through any other available therapeutic procedure."*

A Universal Need for Chelation Therapy

As early as 1968, Dr. Lamar predicted, *"I have little doubt that eventually new ligands (chelating agents) will be created that will be effective by the oral (natural supplements) route.* ***** *That will be the big step that will bring chelation therapy to the reach of any patient suffering from any form of calcific disease, plaque and cholesterol build-up."*

"The great advance in preventive medicine lies in keeping the arteries open and clean BEFORE the symptoms or attack which make the disorder obvious to everybody," Dr. Evers declared. *"This is where chelation therapy has its greatest future."*

There are hundreds of chelation clinics in America and around the world. The best web source of doctors for chelation therapy is ACAM (the American College for Advancement in Medicine), *www.acamnet.org* where you can locate doctors in your area by zip code and also doctors around the world. ACAM address is: 8001 Irvine Center Drive, #825, Irvine, California 92618. They also have a physician referral hotline: 1-800-532-3688.

In Europe, we met with world famous Dr. Claus Martin who has the vision, wisdom and education to direct his lovely *Four Seasons Clinic* in the Bavarian Alps that provides chelation, oxygen, and live cell therapy from March to Nov. These are remarkable life-prolonging treatments that can help reverse the age-related and degenerative cardiovascular diseases. Hollywood Stars, Famous Statesmen and other noteworthy people have and are reaping the benefits of his treatments. He is a long time highly respected member of ACAM. There are over 200 chelation clinics throughout Europe. Checkout ACAM website or if in Europe write or call:

Dr. Claus Martin, M.D., Four Seasons Clinic
Box 244, D-83700 Rottach-Egern, Germany
PHONE: 011-49-8022-26780; FAX 011-49-8022-24740

*Health Stores now have oral chelation supplements and Niacin (B3), etc.

A light, happy heart lives longer. – William Shakespeare

The heart that loves is always young. – Greek proverb

Life is a song, love is the music.

The Benefits of Chelation Therapy*

Chelation Therapy helps halt bad effects of ageing and heart disease and initiates the body's healing process, often reversing the damage. Some of the benefits are:

- **Reduces Free Radical Activity in Blood:** Research shows EDTA can have antioxidant nutrients – vitamins A, C and E, selenium, and amino acid complexes. These not only mop up free radicals but also assist in reinforcing the stability of cell membranes (see pages 24-26).

- **Blocks Calcium Absorption, Repairs Damaged Muscles, Improves the Cell Energy Production:** EDTA removes the toxic metal ions such as lead, calcium, mercury, cadmium, copper, iron, and aluminum from the blood stream. By removing the extra calcium from the blood stream, there is no more free calcium available to produce plaque. It means that the cells can start to repair themselves. Their production of energy increases. As more and more cells rebuild, our body becomes healthier. They can ward off intruders. The result is that we have started a salvage and regeneration activity that repairs previously damaged muscles and heart. And the whole body benefits as a result.

- **Reduces Blood Stickiness or Clotting:** EDTA helps to reduce blood platelet formation. This makes the blood less sticky. The blood can now flow through narrow arteries. It can flow through even partially blocked arteries minimizing the effect of the blockage.

- **Normalizes Abnormal Cholesterol and HDL Levels:** Researchers have found that EDTA infusion, combined with vitamin and mineral supplements, raised the good (HDL) cholesterol and lowered the bad (LDL) cholesterol. If the HDL was low, it was raised; however, if it was already high, its level remains the same. Similarly, the LDL was lowered if it was high. EDTA optimizes the ratio of HDL and LDL.

- **Mental Health:** Researchers have noticed that patients who have undergone chelation treatment are less depressed. They were more alert, alive and happier, and had better concentration, memory and more energy.

198

---

*See web: holisticonline.com/Chelation/chel_benefits.htm

Chapter 20

Herbs – Garlic – Food Supplements
Mother Nature's Healers

This book gives you a healthy lifestyle program for a healthy, rewarding life. When you follow The Bragg Healthy Lifestyle you can build a strong, healthy heart. This will take you down the path to increased health confidence, creativity and vitality! Please remember always strive to live a more healthy, happy, positive life!

In building a healthier and stronger heart don't forget the miraculous healing gifts available from Mother Nature's kingdom. For thousands of years people around the world have used herbs and plants as medicines, tonics and remedies. Many of them are renowned for increasing heart health. Today, scientific research supports the traditional use of many of these medicinal plants. Herbs such as garlic, ginkgo, hawthorn, bilberry, gotu kola and rosemary have been traditionally used and scientifically researched for the treatment of heart and circulatory conditions. Here's a brief description of some of the most effective herbs. In addition to The Bragg Healthy Lifestyle, make use of these miracles of the plant world for your heart's health and fitness. Remember to consult your health care professional before substituting herbs in a previously existing condition. The key to a healthy heart is prevention and The Bragg Healthy Heart Program.

Garlic – The Herb that Lowers Cholesterol

Garlic is one of nature's great miracles. No other medicinal plant is more effective in the treatment and prevention of atherosclerosis! No wonder there has been increased research involving garlic and cardiovascular health. Research shows eating garlic regularly decreases serum cholesterol and dangerous triglyceride levels! People who eat garlic regularly have healthier arteries and blood than those who don't. This is why people in France, Greece, Italy, etc. (who traditionally eat lots of garlic) have a lower incidence of heart attack and disease than people in the United States.

Garlic – Your Body's Health Friend

Garlic's health role in protecting your heart – the cloves contain many natural anticoagulants that help thin the blood and help protect against platelet stickiness – thus lowering risk of clotting and even a stroke! Plus, garlic has potent immune-enhancing properties, it may eradicate many types of bacteria and fungi, including salmonella and candida; as well as inhibit gastrointestinal ulcers. (We love garlic.) See web: *www.garlic-central.com*

In 1993 an extensive revealing study on garlic *(called poor man's penicillin)* in *Annals of Internal Medicine* found small amounts of fresh garlic eaten daily can significantly lower cholesterol levels in people with high cholesterol levels. Other exciting studies show that garlic helps decrease the blood's bad LDL-cholesterol levels while increasing levels of good HDL-cholesterol! It's also a general blood tonic. Please make fresh garlic part of your daily routine – a clove a day for prevention, 2-3 cloves to lower your cholesterol.

Remove garlic's outer papery skin. Let it sit for 10 minutes after chopping, to let the beneficial enzymes develop. Varieties of garlic and onions (red onion is our favorite) are: shallots, elephant garlic, garlic spears, leeks, chives and scallions – all beneficial to your health!

200

The Healing Powers of Onions

Ancient Egyptians and Romans prized the extraordinary healing powers of onions, also garlic. Research supports these claims. According to studies done by nutrition department at Pennsylvania State University, consuming one medium onion a day helps lower your cholesterol by 15 percent. The sulfur compounds in onions help lower dangerous levels of blood fats and help keep plaque from adhering to artery walls. (See web: *onions-usa.org*)

Onions come in many varieties: yellow, red and white. Sweet onions like Vidalia, Maui and Walla Walla have a lower sulfur content than other more pungent varieties. To minimize tears, chill onions for half an hour before peeling and chopping. It's best to eat them raw for their full health benefit in salads, dips, spreads, soups and sandwiches. When cooking onions, lightly sauté them, for over-cooking can destroy important enzymes.

Ginkgo – Improves Blood Flow to Brain

Over the last 40 years, Ginkgo has been one of the most scientifically researched medicinal herbs in the world today. Scientists know that *Gingko Biloba* (leaf) *Extracts* (GBE) dilate arteries, capillaries and veins, which increases blood flow. Therefore GBE reduces blood clotting and clogging of the arteries. GBE's strong cardiovascular benefits are localized in the brain. Increasing evidence supports the GBE effectiveness in treating ailments associated with too little blood flow to the brain (such as short-term memory loss, senility, short attention span and depression). In addition, GBE inhibit platelet aggregation, reduce blood clotting and work through antioxidants to protect our vascular walls from free-radical damage (see pages 24-26). Look for GBE supplements in health stores. See: *ginkgobilobaextract.net*

Hawthorn – Multiple Cardiovascular Benefits

The Hawthorn Berry is used for the treatment of hypertensions, angina, cardiac arrhythmias and congestive heart failure. Scientific studies show hawthorn's ability to dilate blood vessels (especially coronary vessels associated with angina). These effects can be traced to the pigment found in hawthorn flowers, leaves and berries. These phytonutrients include bioflavonoids that have strong antioxidant properties and assist our body in ridding itself of free radicals. They also help our body distribute and effectively use vitamin C and strengthen capillaries. These stronger capillaries and dilated blood vessels allow our heart to better circulate blood, thus delivering oxygen to every system of our body and providing our heart with the nutrients it needs. Also use as a preventative as part of a healthy heart lifestyle.

Ginkgo extract health benefits: *improvement in blood flow to most tissues and organs and protection against oxidative cell damage from free radicals.*

Hawthorn Berry: *Laboratory studies show that this herb has antioxidant properties that help protect against the formation of plaques, which leads atherosclerosis. Plaque buildup in the vessels that supply the heart with oxygen-rich blood may cause chest pain (angina) and heart attacks while plaque buildup in the arteries that supply blood to the brain may result in stroke.*
– herbwisdom.com/herb-hawthorn-berry.html

Cayenne – Lifesaver for Heart & Circulation

People worldwide use a variety of hot peppers in their cooking. Peppers are also firmly rooted in traditions of folk medicine. When we talk of cayenne pepper, we are referring to red hot peppers of the genus, *capsicum annuum* – which includes cayenne, the famous Tabasco pepper, Mexican chili peppers, pimiento, the Louisiana long pepper and others. All contain pungent *capsaicin,* that gives hot pepper its kick and important healthy active ingredients for your circulation and heart.

Prior to the Civil War the red pepper had gained a reputation in the U.S. as a heat rub when applied to the skin. Since then people have found that it promotes health and healing in many ways! Example: cayenne has become popular as a digestive aid and a pain reliever salve for sprains, backaches, etc. For arthritis, osteoarthritis, joint pain and stiffness, also try glucosamine, chondroitin and MSM combo. These help heal, regenerate and soothe. Also try cayenne and DMSO lotions (pat lightly – don't rub).

Cayenne is a powerful heart and health healer, so make use of it's potential! Studies confirm cayenne's effect as a general blood tonic, linking it to a reduction of blood clotting. These studies show capsaicin (cayenne) has beneficial effects on the cardiovascular system, helps lowers cholesterol levels and helps prevent heart disease, see pages 19 and 222. For healthy heart benefits add cayenne flakes to food regularly to season: soups, potatoes, vegetables, salads, beans, rice, etc. instead of salt! I take one cayenne capsule (40,000 HU) daily with meals. Try broth: stir $1/2$ lemon, 1 tsp. Bragg Aminos, tiny pinch cayenne flakes in a cup of hot water. See web: *healingdaily.com/detoxification-diet/cayenne.htm*

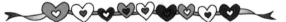

A recent Japanese study has linked cayenne (capsaicin) intake with improved oxygen levels in the blood. This helps keep your heart and cardiovascular system open and your brain and memory more alert. (I take a 40,000 HU (heat units) capsule of cayenne daily. – PB)

Herbs & Supplements for Healthy Heart: *Cayenne powder & tincture, Hawthorn Berry tinctures, Gotu Kola extracts, Evening Primrose Oil, Motherwort, Magnesium, Red Sage, Cinnamon, Gingko Biloba, Omega 3 fish or flax oils, Chromium Picolinate, Licorice Root Tea, Vitamin E, Selenium & CoQ10.*
– Linda Page, N.D., Ph.D., *Healthy Healing* (www.healthyhealing.com)

B-Vitamins Important for Healthy Heart

Evidence shows certain B-vitamins help reduce the risk of heart disease by lowering the harmful amino acid *homocysteine* from the blood (It's not in Bragg Aminos). Too much homocysteine brings damage to cells lining blood vessel walls. Harvard study shows B vitamins (B1, B3 *niacin*, B5 *pantothenic acid*, B6, B12 and folic acid) reduce homocysteine levels in the blood. This is especially important for those who are at risk for cardiovascular problems, because 1 in every 3 people with cardiovascular disease have dangerously high levels of homocysteine. See pages 45 and 222. See web: *www.homocysteine.com*

Plant foods are major sources of vitamin B6 and folic acid. However, vitamin B12 is not found in vegetables. Vegetarians can obtain sufficient B12 from tofu and other soybean products; or from vitamin supplements. We recommend Bragg Nutrition Yeast – a delicious flavor enhancer rich in B-vitamins (even B12). Bragg Nutritional Yeast is great for pets too! (Helps keep fleas away.) We sprinkle it over salads, soups, veggies, potatoes, tofu, rice, beans, etc. and popcorn. See our delicious popcorn recipe on page 140.

Folic Acid Helps Protect the Blood

Folic acid plays a vital role in the smooth functioning of a healthy body. Revered as a brain food, it's needed for growth of red and white blood cells and the body's energy production. Deficiencies of folic acid, B6 and B12 can lead to serious conditions such as depression, insomnia, immune system problems and dangerously high homocysteine levels.

In addition to supplements, folic acid is found in dates, Bragg Nutritional Yeast, broccoli, etc. (see more next page). Folic acid works best taken with vitamin C, B6 and B12.

Two must-read books by Kilmer S. McCully, M.D. *Homocysteine Revolution* and *Heart Revolution* (*Amazon.com*) educate the reader about the deadly toxic effects of high homocysteine levels and tragic results to cardiovascular system.

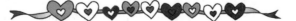

People who don't get enough folic acid to metabolize harmful homocysteine have 3x the risk of a heart attack as those who do. The higher the level of homocysteine in the body, the greater the risk of blockage in a person's carotid arteries.

Healthy Food Sources of Folic Acid*

– The Health Nutrient Bible, LYNN SONBERG

Food Source	mgs
Spinach, (raw or steamed) 1 Cup	262
Asparagus, (raw or steamed) 1 Cup	176
Lima beans, (raw or steamed) 1 Cup	156
Broccoli, (raw or steamed) 1 Cup	108
Wheat germ, 1/4 Cup	106
Beets, (raw or steamed) 1 Cup	90
Cauliflower, (raw or steamed) 1 Cup	64
Orange (navel), 1 medium	47
Cantaloupe, 1/2 melon	46
Cabbage, (raw or steamed) 1 Cup	40
Tofu, firm 1/2 Cup	37

Other healthy food sources of Folic Acid are: green leafy vegetables, black-eyed peas, sunflower seeds, kidney beans, and winter squash

Vitamin C is for Capillaries and Cholesterol

For your capillary health, turn to vitamin C. Thousands of studies conclude vitamin C makes healthier capillaries by reducing clotting in the bloodstream. Remember, your blood must move along your capillaries in single file, cell by cell. A blood clot can completely stop the flow of blood through these microscopic vessels! Researchers recently attributed other cardiovascular benefits to C, including clearing of cholesterol and calcium from arterial walls. It's a strong weapon against hardening and clogging of your arteries. Taken before bedtime, studies show it prevents heart attacks during sleep and in the morning. This new info supports studies conducted 40 years ago by pioneering Doctor G. C. Willis, whose patients showed improvements of arteriosclerosis in leg arteries, etc. when given 500 mg. vitamin C, 3 times daily. We daily get at least 3,000 mg. of mixed vitamin C (with rutin and bioflavonoids) and Quercetin in supplements and fresh citrus fruits, green leafy vegetables, tomatoes and in the many fruits and vegetables we eat.

Godfrey Oakley, M.D., of the Centers for Disease Control and Prevention, says there is strong evidence from over 200 studies that increased consumption of Folic Acid (from foods or supplements) helps prevent cardiovascular disease.

Vitamin C is one of many antioxidants. Vitamin E and beta-carotene are two other well-known antioxidants. Antioxidants are nutrients that block some of the damage caused by free radicals. – nlm.nih.gov/medlineplus.htm

Vitamin E – Essential For Heart Health

According to Canada's Pioneer Shute brothers and scientist Dr. Richard Passwater, we all need vitamin E for the general health and proper body functioning. It's an essential vitamin for cardiovascular health. A low vitamin E level in the blood is one of the most reliable warning indicators of heart disease risk and future cardiovascular problems. See web: *vitaminefacts.org*

Why is vitamin E essential? It prevents damage by free radicals formed when fat is exposed to oxygen and heat. Vitamin E protects the arteries by neutralizing oxidized cholesterol. It helps prevent the red blood cells from clumping together, dissolves blood clots and increases oxygenation of blood, which improves the heart's supply of oxygen. Vitamin E dilates the capillaries, improves capillary strength and helps protect against cardiovascular scarring after a heart attack. It also helps provide relief from complaints of poor circulation, like leg cramps, cold feet, hands, etc. We recommend a daily allowance of 400 to 800 IU's of natural mixed-tocopherol. In addition to supplements, there's significant quantities vitamin E in wheat germ, cold-pressed vegetable oils, organic whole grains, dark leafy green vegetables, beans, raw nuts and seeds – our favorite, sunflower seeds.

E Tocotrienols: New Kids on the Block

These compounds demonstrate vitamin E-like activity, with added protection benefits that help with serious heart problems: they help lower cholesterol and there's evidence E Tocotrienols provide greater antioxidant protection against lipid peroxidation than standard vitamin E. New E Tocotrienols can be purchased in health stores as a single supplement – or as part of the vitamin E with mixed E Tocopherols. See web: *lifeextension.com*

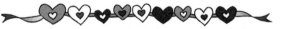

Vitamin E helps prevent breakdown of body tissues. – HealingDaily.com

Vitamin C and E are powerful antioxidants and play a critical role in heart health. Vitamin E is also an anticoagulant that helps keep blood platelets from clumping together so they can easily go through small capillaries. Vitamin E also protects arterial walls from free-radical damage. – Dr. Julian Whitaker

Beta-Carotene Protects Against Heart Disease

Beta carotene plays an extremely important part in promoting heart health. More than 200 studies have confirmed that foods rich in flavonoids, carotenoids and other antioxidants can reduce risk of numerous health conditions, including heart health and a stronger immune system. Beta-carotene is transformed in the body into vitamin A, which helps protect against heart disease in several ways. The most important is its ability to neutralize the toxic free radicals (see pages 24-26).

What is beta-carotene? Beta-carotene is probably the most well known of the carotenoids, a phytonutrients family (see page 114) that represents one of the most widespread groups of naturally occurring pigments. It is known as "pro-vitamin A" compound, able to convert into retinol, an active form of vitamin A. In recent years, beta-carotene has received a tremendous amount of attention as a potential anti-cancer and anti-aging compound. Beta-carotene is a powerful antioxidant, protecting the cells of the body from damage caused by free radicals.

206

You should not take high-dose supplements of beta-carotene alone, but get it in combination with your diet. Food sources of beta-carotene include sweet potatoes, carrots, spinach, turnip greens, winter squash, collard greens, cilantro and fresh thyme. To maximize availability of carotenoids in foods listed below, some should be eaten raw in salads, steamed lightly or baked.

Healthy Food Sources of Beta Carotene

Food Source	mcgs
Pumpkin – bake or steam (1 cup)	17,003
Sweet Potatoes – bake or steam (1 cup)	13,308
Carrots – fresh, slice or grate (1 cup)	10,605
Turnip greens – steam & drain (1 cup)	6,588
Kale – raw, chop (1 cup)	6,181
Butternut squash – raw, grate (1 cup)	5,916
Cantaloupe – fresh, dice (1 cup)	3,151
Spinach – raw, chop (1 cup)	1,688
Mango – fresh, dice (1 cup)	734
Apricot – fresh (1)	383

Magnesium For Your Heart, Blood & Arteries

Magnesium provides many benefits for your heart health. It reduces blood pressure and controls the skipping heart. It relaxes the muscles of the artery walls and improves blood flow. Magnesium helps shuttle potassium in and out of cells, maintaining proper membrane balance (homeostasis). It acts like a calcium channel blocker to stabilize cardiac conduction, heart muscle and vascular membranes. Please be alert to the importance of magnesium. It keeps heart, blood and arteries working together. Deficiencies in this essential mineral are often the root of many cardiovascular problems. Though magnesium naturally occurs in most raw foods, a healthy daily amount of 250 mg. is hard to attain eating processed foods. Eat organic apples, apricots, avocados, bananas, green leafy vegetables, garlic, beans, soybeans, soy products, raw nuts and seeds, brown rice, tofu, whole wheat and other whole grains, which are rich in magnesium. Herbs such as cayenne, alfalfa, fennel, hops, paprika and others add magnesium for your heart's health! See web: *all-natural.com/bone.html.*

Magnesium is vital to your health and enzymatic activity. A deficiency can interfere with nerves and muscle impulses. When that happens, your blood pressure, heart activity and circulatory flow can be affected. Side-effects can lead to high blood pressure, cardiac arrhythmia, cardiac arrest and stress damage in arterial walls! For arrhythmia, magnesium orotate works miracles, along with calcium.

Calcium: The Other Half of the Dynamic Duo

Calcium is important too, because of its synergistic relationship with magnesium. Although most people associate calcium deficits with poor bone health, low levels can also increase your vulnerability to high blood pressure. But you must be careful about the amount of calcium you take. More than 2,000 mg of calcium per day can cause your kidneys to excrete magnesium!

Magnesium is a superstar nutrient that plays a role in approximately 300 functions in the body. – Life Extension Magazine (www.lef.org)

Take 1,000 mg daily of calcium in conjunction with 500 mg daily of magnesium. Postmenopausal women are advised to take 1,500 mg of calcium. Choose a calcium formula that contains mixed compounds such as citrate, carbonate, aspartate and gluconate in combination with similar magnesium complex. – see: drsinatra.com

Locations in the Body Where Osteoporosis, Arthritis, Pain and Misery Hit the Hardest

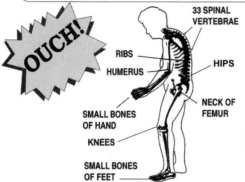

OUCH!

33 SPINAL VERTEBRAE
RIBS
HUMERUS
HIPS
NECK OF FEMUR
SMALL BONES OF HAND
KNEES
SMALL BONES OF FEET

OSTEOPOROSIS
Affects over 30 Million and Kills 400,000 Americans Annually

Boron
Miracle Trace Mineral For Healthy Bones

208

BORON – A trace mineral for healthier bones that also helps the body absorb more vital calcium, minerals and necessary hormones! Good sources are most vegetables, fresh and sun- dried fruits, prunes, raw nuts, soybeans and Bragg Nutritional Yeast.

The U.S. Department of Agriculture's Human Nutrition Lab in Grand Forks, North Dakota, says boron is usually found in soil and in foods, but many Americans eat a diet low in boron. They conducted a 17 week study which showed a daily 3 to 6 mgs. boron supplement enabled participants to reduce loss (demineralization) of calcium, phosphorus and magnesium from their bodies. This loss is usually caused by eating processed fast foods and lots of meat, salt, sugar and fat and a dietary lack of fresh organic vegetables, fruits and whole grains. (See web: *all-natural.com*)

After 8 weeks on boron, participants' calcium loss was cut 40%. It also helped double important hormone levels vital in maintaining calcium and healthy bones. Millions of women on estrogen replacement therapy for osteoporosis* may want to use boron as a healthier choice. Also consider natural progesterone (2%) raw yam cream. For pain, joint support and healing use a glucosamine/chondroitin/MSM combo (*caps, liquid or roll-on*).

Scientific studies show women benefit from healthy lifestyle that includes some gentle (vitamin D3) sunshine and ample exercise (*even weight lifting*) to maintain healthier bones, combined with a low-fat, high-fiber, carbohydrate, and fresh fruits, salads, sprouts, greens and vegetable diet. This lifestyle helps protect against heart disease, high blood pressure, cancer and many other ailments. I'm happy to see science now agrees with my Dad who first stated these health truths in the 1930's.

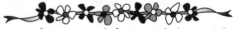

*For more hormone and osteoporosis facts read pioneer John Lee, M.D.'s book – What Your Doctor May Not Tell You About Menopause. (amazon.com)

Potassium Helps Strengthen the Heart

The heart is a large muscle and your master pump. It uses large amounts of potassium to keep going strong and healthy, hour after hour, for your entire life! It is the hardest working muscle in the body. The heart must have a constant, continuous supply of power and energy to continue beating! Apple cider vinegar contains natural potassium that combines with healthy heart foods to make the heart muscle stronger and also help to normalize blood pressure and cholesterol.

Take an extra 1/2 tsp of Bragg Raw Organic Apple Cider Vinegar (ACV) in 1/2 glass distilled/purified water, twice daily between meals – good before exercise. But also enjoy your basic 3 ACV cocktail drinks daily (see page 140).

Potassium is the Master Mineral

Potassium is an essential mineral for the body because it puts toxic poisons in solution so they can be flushed out of the body. **The body is self-cleansing, self-correcting, self-repairing and self-healing!** Just give it the tools to work with and you will have a painless, tireless, ageless body, regardless of age! Forget calendar years, for age is not toxic! You age prematurely when you suffer from potassium deficiencies and malnutrition! This low Vital Force and waste buildup (poor elimination) allows disease to proliferate.*

The Bragg Healthy Lifestyle helps you rebuild your Vital Force (more on Vital Force in our *Nerve Force* Book see pages 249-251). Watch the transformation that takes place in your body when you faithfully follow ACV regime. You can, and will create the kind of person you want to be! It's exciting to plan, plot and follow through!

Although you must follow this program closely, do not try to do everything listed here immediately. Remember, it took you a long time of living by wrong habits to cause any of the problems your body might have now. So, it's going to take time for the body to cleanse, repair and rebuild itself into a more *perfect health home* for you! Please remember, your body is your temple while on this earth – so cherish it and protect it!

---

*See the website: healthcentral.com

Essential Fatty Acids Save Lives

Omega-3 and omega-6 essential fatty acids (EFA) are vital components of cell membranes. The omega-3 fatty acid, found in fish oil, is important for patients with heart disease. This fatty acid can affect the body's immune system, inflammatory response, blood flow, blood pressure and coagulability of the blood. Omega-3 fatty acids can have a marked effect on reducing the triglyceride levels.

Studies confirm omega-3 fatty acids in fish and flax oil provides tremendous protection from heart disease. They aid in the stabilization of the heart's electrical activity reducing risk of fatal arrhythmias and sudden cardiac death. Almost all fresh, raw, unprocessed nuts, grains and seeds contain substantial quantities of the omega-6 fatty acids. Fish oil and flaxseed are the most abundant sources of omega-3 fatty acids.

HEALTHY OILS RICH IN OMEGA-3 & OMEGA-6
Good for the heart & delicious on salads, greens & veggies.

	Omega-3	Omega-6
Flax Seed	57%	16%
Pumpkin	15%	42%
Soy	9%	50%
Walnut	5%	51%

L-Arginine – Essential to Heart Health

L-Arginine is an amino acid that has shown promise in prevention of atherosclerosis. It is thought to be the primary source for production of nitrogen molecules involved in maintaining elasticity of blood vessels. Research has shown that L-Arginine may be helpful for people with high cholesterol. (Bragg Liquid Aminos contains this very important amino acid. See page 252 for more info).

To increase your omega-3 intake try flaxseeds (page 119) and walnuts. $^1/_4$ cup flaxseeds contains about 7 grams of omega-3 fatty acids, while $^1/_4$ cup walnuts contains about 2.3 grams. Add this nut-seed combination to salads, baked potatoes, trail mix, granola, etc. Other omega-3 sources: fish, squash and olive oil. (Use Bragg's Organic Extra-Virgin Cold Pressed – don't hi-fry, only lightly saute with it.) Adding 2 Tbsps flaxseeds daily to diet, you will be close to recommended 4 grams of omega-3.

Strokes result when blood clots form in the arteries, blocking nutrients to brain cells. Omega 3 fish oils are anticoagulants present in fish such as tuna or salmon. You can also get a good dose in our favorite daily teaspoon of flaxseed oil or ground flax seeds (page 119). Onions and garlic are other natural anticoagulants.

Ubiquinol CoQ10 Combats Heart Disease, Cancer, Gum Disease and Ageing

Ubiquinol Coenzyme Q10, a potent improved antioxidant that protects cells from free radicals, also is involved in energy production in cells. Although made by every body cell, production diminishes with age and disease.

The heart is one of the few body organs to function continuously without resting; therefore, the heart muscle requires highest energetic support. Any condition that causes a decrease in CoQ10 could impair heart's energetic capacity, thus leaving heart tissues more susceptible to free radical attack! In long term studies, Ubiquinol CoQ10, was found to prolong life by years, (100 mg. am and 50 mg. early evening). In some patients, the disease was eliminated completely. Peter H. Langsjoen, MD, cardiologist co-authored study found patients reduced their heart and blood pressure medications by 40-50% and 25% of his patients became drug-free (web: *lef.org*).

Oligomeric Proanthocyanidins (OPCs)

You've probably heard about the benefits of red wine, green tea (caffeine free), and grape juice. All are in the family of oligomeric proanthocyanidins (OPCs). OPCs are flavonoid complexes, found in most plants and a part of the human diet. They are found in large quantities in grape seed extract and grape skins, in red grapes, in the red skins of peanuts, in coconuts and apples. These free radical scavengers are quickly absorbed into the bloodstream where they cross the blood/brain barrier. OPCs may help protect against the effects of internal and environmental stresses such as cigarette smoking and pollution, as well as supporting normal body metabolic processes. The effects may include depressing blood fat, softening the blood vessels, lowering blood pressure, preventing blood vessel sclerosis, dropping blood viscosity and preventing blood clot formation.

Additionally, studies have shown that OPCs may prevent cardiovascular diseases by counteracting the negative effects of high cholesterol on the heart and blood vessels. See front inside cover for more information.

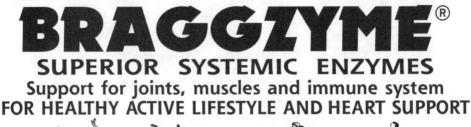

BRAGGZYME®

SUPERIOR SYSTEMIC ENZYMES
Support for joints, muscles and immune system
FOR HEALTHY ACTIVE LIFESTYLE AND HEART SUPPORT

Dr. Paul C. Bragg, Health Pioneer, was the first to introduce enzyme supplements in Health Stores in 1931. Now Bragg Health Science Formulas is proud to introduce most advanced systemic enzyme supplement available today. BRAGGZYME the Superior Systemic Enzyme is an all natural superior systemic fibrinolytic enzyme that contains powerful 500mg Complex (Nattokinase, Serrapeptase, Bromelain, Papain, Protease and Lipase), with 4,500 Fibrinolytic Units (FU) per capsule.

"Good Circulation is Key to A Healthy Body!" – Paul C. Bragg, ND, PhD.

This exclusive systemic enzyme blend provides nutritional and cardiovascular support you need to help maintain a normal inflammatory response and maintain safe normal fibrin levels for a healthy cardiovascular system.* Braggzyme contains no animal derivatives, no artificial flavors, no artificial coloring, no yeast and no wheat.

- Enzyme support for back, joint, muscle, tendon and immune health system.*
- Boost energy levels – infuses life-giving oxygen to every cell in your body.*
- Nutritional support to help maintain a normal inflammatory response.*
- Helps eliminate dangerous fibrin levels for a healthier blood flow.*
- Helps keep your hands, feet and the entire body warm.*
- Helps improve and keep memory and brain sharp.*
- Contains no animal derivatives, no yeast, no wheat, no artificial flavors and no artificial colors.
- Kosher Certified
- 100% Safe, All Natural Veg. Formula in Veg. Cap

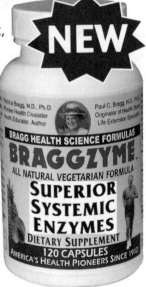

NEW

* These statements have not been evaluated by the Food and Drug Administration. This product is not intended to diagnose, treat, cure, or prevent any disease.

"I have been taking Braggzyme for the last several months, and have felt a major improvement in my knee pain caused by sports, snowboarding, etc. Thanks, Braggzyme!"
– Brian Evans, Manager, Lassens Natural Foods, Santa Barbara, CA

My doctor said that elevated fibrinogen levels are associated with an increased risk of heart attack and strokes because it can promote formation of dangerous blood clots. Good news! I've been taking Braggzyme and my blood fibrinogen level was 329 and it came down 50 points, now it's a safe 279.
– Kathy Duerr, Portland, OR

Since I have been on Braggzyme, I have tremendous energy and now no more body aches and pains! My memory is sharper and I am enjoying vibrant energy. Thanks to Braggzyme. – Robert DeCastro, California

Chapter 21

Heart Healthy Programs

While outlining our Heart Fitness Program we have told you in detail about the vicious enemies of the heart. Know your enemies and keep away from them! If you have lived a haphazard life and have damaged your heart, we believe that you can still make a comeback and build a healthy heart for yourself. Remember that your body is self-cleansing, repairing and healing! Given the chance, it will do its best to rebuild a vigorous heart for you. But you must work with your body – not against it!

Do not be discouraged if you have an ailing or damaged heart. Faithfully following our program of clean, natural living will help you to live out your entire natural life span! Yes, your miraculous body possesses tremendous recuperative powers which – if fully used – are of great help even in the most serious cases of heart trouble.

BRAGG Healthy Heart Fitness Pointers

♥ A vegetarian diet is healthier. Instead of meat, eat unsaturated vegetarian proteins – such as soybeans, tofu, beans, raw seeds and nuts such as: sunflower, sesame, flaxseed, pumpkin, almonds, pecans, and walnuts.

♥ Use no salt – toss the salt shaker! (Use Bragg Liquid Aminos, Bragg Sprinkle (24 herbs & spices) and Kelp.

♥ Eat no dairy products – milk, cheese, butter – high in clogging, saturated fats. (Use soy, almond, rice milk products.)

♥ If you want to eat eggs, limit it to 3 or 4 a week. Organically fed, free-range chicken eggs are healthiest.

♥ Fruits and vegetables – organic, raw or lightly steamed or cooked – should form 60% to 70% of your diet.

♥ Don't use any white sugars or the toxic commercial substitutes such as aspartame, NutraSweet, etc. – they contain harmful chemicals (see page 62).

♥ Fast 24 hour period weekly (pages 147-154). This gives heart and vital organs physiological rest. It will also help reduce cholesterol and toxins in the body and arteries.

♥ A low-fat diet, ample exercise and brisk walking with deep breathing helps you keep cholesterol levels normal.

- Absolutely no smoking or drinking alcohol.

- Get plenty of recharging sleep and peaceful relaxation.

- Don't let anybody or anything put undue pressure on you. Worry, stress, and tension do not necessarily cause a heart attack – but they don't help you avoid it either!

- Eat healthy, simple, natural, organic foods and products.

- Eat slowly and chew your food thoroughly. Chewing is the first process in digestion. Saying grace helps digestion!

- Don't over-eat – it burdens your body and causes obesity.

- Get plenty of regular exercise. Although complete rest may be necessary just after an acute heart attack or when the heart is very weak. When this stage is past you will find regular daily exercise a great help in rebuilding and revitalizing the heart and circulation.

- Don't get into emotional arguments, they waste precious nervous energy! Walk away from unpleasant people and situations – it's best to avoid them completely!

- Get the Happiness Habit! A cheerful, happy disposition helps promote health, happiness and longevity.

- Keep away from all artificial stimulants – coffee, china tea (caffeine), soda/cola drinks and alcohol. Do not let anyone tell you that alcohol will help your heart.

- Walk! Breathe deeply and enjoy daily brisk walks!

Follow BRAGG's Heart Fitness Program

Would you trust the repair of your car to someone who had no knowledge of automobiles? Of course not! It is never too late to obtain and apply health knowledge. We have already described to you the structure and functioning of your precious heart and circulatory system and explained the importance of keeping the blood cholesterol at a healthy normal level. We suggest that you reread this book from time to time. Let this Program be your Faithful Guide on the Highway to Super Health.

Stress and emotional turmoil can cause or worsen high blood pressure. Reduce stress through regular exercise, which should be a part of your lifestyle, to lower blood pressure and improve heart health. – Health and Nutrition Breakthrough

Mother Nature cannot be rushed – but if you cooperate with her, you can have *the heart of a lion.* If you have a weak heart or weak *pipes* that are clogged, remember that it took a long time to get them into that condition. Be patient with Mother Nature while the regeneration, rejuvenation and cleansing processes take place within your body.

A fit, youthful heart can be yours, if you are willing to work for it! No one else can make your heart strong. It depends entirely on you. Your eating habits, your daily lifestyle and your physical activity will determine the condition of your heart and the health you will enjoy.

Dr. John Harvey Kellogg's Famous Vegetarian Diet for Heart Patients

Dr. John Harvey Kellogg was the founder and director of the great Battle Creek Sanitarium at Battle Creek, Michigan. Sick people from all over the world – even royalty – traveled there to be under his personal care. My father was fortunate enough to work with him.

As soon as a heart attack victim was brought to the Sanitarium, Dr. Kellogg would put them on a strict vegetarian diet with the advice that this should be a lifetime diet. It was a strict, exclusively vegetarian regime consisting of fruit, vegetables, seeds and nuts. No meat, no fish, no eggs, no dairy products, no coffee, no alcohol and no salt were allowed. Dr. Kellogg believed this strict vegetarian diet was the only one which a heart sufferer should eat because it contained absolutely no cholesterol. It was also a salt-free diet. The only drinks allowed were herb teas, fresh fruit and vegetable juices and distilled water. Dr. Kellogg told Dad that people who had come to him with serious heart damage had lived as many as 50 additional years on this strict vegetarian diet.

Dr. Kellogg himself lived and practiced until he was well into his 90's He was a strict lacto-vegetarian, eating only a small amount of natural cheese and 3 eggs weekly with the otherwise completely vegetarian diet which he advocated for his heart patients. At age 92 he was still performing delicate operations at his Sanitarium. Today a great many doctors and nutritionists have joined him in recommending a vegetarian diet for all heart patients. See the following pages for Dr. Kellogg's menu ideas.

Dr. Kellogg's Famous Menus:

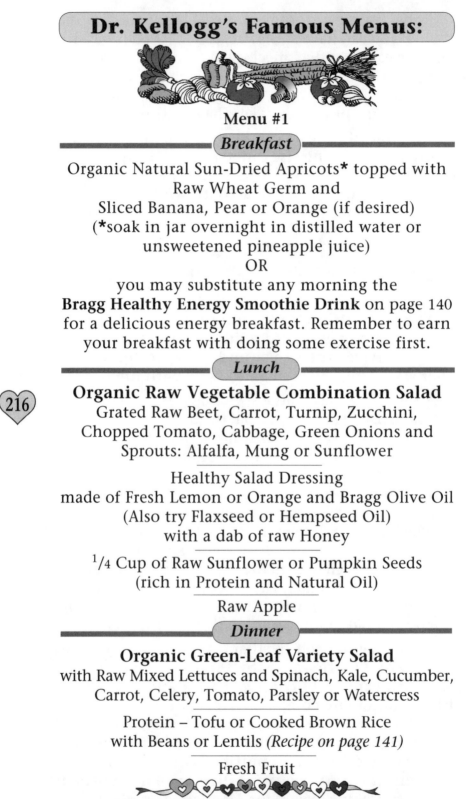

Menu #1

Breakfast

Organic Natural Sun-Dried Apricots* topped with
Raw Wheat Germ and
Sliced Banana, Pear or Orange (if desired)
(*soak in jar overnight in distilled water or
unsweetened pineapple juice)
OR
you may substitute any morning the
Bragg Healthy Energy Smoothie Drink on page 140
for a delicious energy breakfast. Remember to earn
your breakfast with doing some exercise first.

Lunch

216

Organic Raw Vegetable Combination Salad
Grated Raw Beet, Carrot, Turnip, Zucchini,
Chopped Tomato, Cabbage, Green Onions and
Sprouts: Alfalfa, Mung or Sunflower

Healthy Salad Dressing
made of Fresh Lemon or Orange and Bragg Olive Oil
(Also try Flaxseed or Hempseed Oil)
with a dab of raw Honey

$1/4$ Cup of Raw Sunflower or Pumpkin Seeds
(rich in Protein and Natural Oil)

Raw Apple

Dinner

Organic Green-Leaf Variety Salad
with Raw Mixed Lettuces and Spinach, Kale, Cucumber,
Carrot, Celery, Tomato, Parsley or Watercress

Protein – Tofu or Cooked Brown Rice
with Beans or Lentils *(Recipe on page 141)*

Fresh Fruit

Organic apples daily helps keep the doctor away!

Dr. Kellogg's Famous Menus:

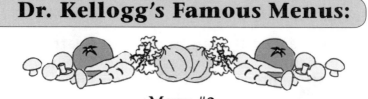

Menu #2

Breakfast

Apple Sauce*
Steel Cut Oats– hot cereal**
served with Honey, Blackstrap Molasses,
Pure Maple Syrup or Stevia (page 60)
100% Whole Wheat or Rye Toast
(*Make your own Apple Sauce, if desired add Honey)
(**Top and serve with Sliced Ripe Banana or other Fruit)

Lunch

Organic Raw Vegetable Combination Salad
(Same as 1st Day)
Vegetable Soup with Natural Barley and Lentils
Whole Rye Toast or Oat Bran - Raisin Muffin

217

Dinner

Cabbage, Apple & Carrot Coleslaw with Spring Onions
Brown Rice or Baked Potato with Skin
Baked or Steamed Carrots and Peas
Fresh Fruit
OR
Avocado, Red Onion and Tomato Salad
Steamed Asparagus or Broccoli
Raw Nuts and Seeds of any kind
Fresh Fruit

*"There is but one way to live and that is
Mother Nature's and God's Healthy Way!"*

Nutrition directly affects growth, development, reproduction, well-being and the physical and mental condition of individuals. Health depends upon nutrition more than on any other single factor. – Dr. William H. Sebrell, Jr.

Studies show both beta-carotene and vitamin C, abundantly found in fruits & vegetables, play vital roles in preventing heart disease & cancers.

Enjoy Positive Thinking and Positive Action

To have a healthy and powerful heart you must develop strong willpower. You must overcome all negative thoughts about the *inevitable* impacts that age supposedly ravages on the heart and body. Do not let cowards and weaklings influence you away from following this Healthy Heart Fitness Program! These fear mongers will try to impart their fear to you by telling you to go easy on exercise, fasting and life changes. Don't believe them! Have faith in your body's ability to improve!

When following this Bragg Healthy Heart Fitness Program and lifestyle you are working with Science and Mother Nature. Don't let unqualified people influence or deter you! Years of health research and investigation have gone into the development of this Heart Fitness Program in order to provide you with a master plan for building a strong, fit heart for a long, fulfilled, healthy life.

Six Points to a Healthy Heart

218

We bring you this book not so much to help you as to help you help yourself! If we repeat certain points, it is with the zeal with which one taps a nail already driven home. Our main objective is to inspire you to a more intense enthusiasm for living The Bragg Healthy Lifestyle and to warn you against certain dangers which you may easily overlooked. Throughout this book we have strongly stressed these six important points to faithfully follow:

1. You have but one heart and one life – you should faithfully take care of these priceless treasures!
2. Your body must obey the commands of your mind, for flesh is dumb and needs a strong health captain!
3. Every bad habit that weakens your heart and shortens your life must be broken and then banished forever!
4. You should demand of yourself a higher living standard for more health, peace of mind and happiness!
5. You should regard your body (your temple) as you would a fine instrument or precision machine whose care and control is in your capable hands!
6. You must draw closer to Mother Nature and God so as to keep your life simple as 1, 2, 3 as your years increase!

Let us, then throw ourselves into Their loving and understanding arms! Try to understand and follow Their wise laws and live as They wants us to live – in superb health for a long, active life of helping this world to be a better, safer, healthier place for us all.

The Complete Naturalist

The complete naturalist's healthy goal is to identify so completely with Mother Nature, that self and the world become one. To do this, keep your life simple as 1, 2, 3, filled with peace, joy and love. Then with serene, clear-eyed confidence put yourself into Mother Nature's and God's hands to run your machine, heal your hurts and comfort you in sickness and adversity. When your time and usefulness on Earth is ended, you'll be called home for eternity in heaven. Psalm 23 is soothing and positive!

Let your body be nourished by natural food, pure distilled (rain) water, fresh air and gentle sunlight. Exercise and relax your body and let Mother Nature do the rest! Treat your body with the same care and wisdom that you would a champion animal. Surely as your animal will take prizes, so will you! Some sneer at health-minded, back-to-nature people. We who believe in God and Mother Nature will enjoy long, happier, healthy, fulfilled lives!

Get Close to Mother Earth and God

It is good to establish contact with Mother Earth, her soil, water, air and sun. Let your bare feet grip into the soft grass or to feel soft mud or sand and squish it between your toes! We love gentle sun (before 10 a.m. or after 3 p.m.) and air baths with few clothes on. We love exercising, stretching, walking and swimming on the beach beside a sea, lake or river. Keep in close touch with Mother Earth and God, letting Their strength and virtue pass into you through your skin and bare feet! *Modern living can complicate our lives with hot house living conditions!* Man was a healthier, happier creature when he lived simpler and closer to Mother Nature.

A healthy body is a guest-chamber for the soul & a sick body is a prison.
– Francis Bacon, English Lord Chancellor, Natural Philosopher (1561-1626),

When you aren't religious or spiritual, at times in life you realize when your life gets hectic and out of control, it's then that you seek a higher power.

Just stand on any big city street and watch the people rushing past. You will see that 3 out of 4 of them are probably sick, obese or physically unfit. Very rarely do you see a super healthy person! Don't be like the average sick or half-sick person. They have never known the real thrill of healthy living! Most people today are addicted to some kind of chemical substance such as tobacco, coffee, tea, alcohol, cola drinks and even some drugs. People turn to drugs when their vitality hits bottom. When health is gone, vitality goes with it and the zest for living. These lost souls turn to drugs in an effort to get false *thrills and kicks* out of life.

Follow the Laws of Mother Nature and God

In the past it was the middle-aged and older people who felt they had to seek drugs or other artificial means to hang onto life. Now, tragically, young people are using drugs of all kinds. They are throwing away their natural vitality and turning their backs on Mother Nature. Now youths have become candidates for heart attacks. The heart is damaged by these stimulants and depressants.

The further we get away from living according to The Laws of Mother Nature and God, then the sicker we get physically, mentally, emotionally and spiritually.

One of the dominant themes of this book is the idea that building a powerful heart at any age is a gradual return to a more natural form of living. Use natural healthy foods, vigorous exercise, deep breathing, restful sleeping, loose fitted clothing and beautiful simplicity of life to reach a closeness to Mother Nature and God that makes you almost one with Them! You will never have a weak, sick heart if you live close and follow in partnership with Them! When you can feel the same strong, pure, elemental forces that manifest themselves in a pine tree expressing themselves in you, then you are on your way to positive, strong health principles.

Begin to live as Mother Nature and God want you to live. Try to feel that They claim you and that you are part of all the glad and growing things on this Good Earth! Put yourself into Mother Nature's and God's hands. We are all eager to aid you on the path to Supreme Health!

Dr. Linda Page's Healthy Heart Program*

Heart disease is still the biggest killer of Americans. A million of us die each year because of heart problems. Yet, most heart disease is 100% preventable with changes in diet and lifestyle. Natural Therapies are proving to reduce mortality better than aggressive medical intervention or even the most advanced drug treatment.

Dr. Linda Page's Diet & Superfoods Therapy

- Your diet is your greatest asset in preventing heart disease. A healthy heart diet has plenty of magnesium and potassium rich foods: fresh greens, sea foods and sea greens; flavonoids from pitted fruits, green herb teas, soy, brown rice, whole grains, garlic and onions.

- Reduce saturated fat to no more than 10% of your daily calorie intake. Especially limit fats from animal sources and hydrogenated oils. Wisely pay conscious attention to avoiding red meats, caffeine products, refined sugars, fatty, salty and fried foods, prepared meats and soft drinks! The rewards are worth the effort.

- Eat 70% of daily calories from complex carbohydrates like vegetables and grains; 20% from low fat protein sources. Vitamin C-rich foods – tomatoes, citrus juice and apple cider vinegar greatly enhance iron absorption.

- Eat less than 100mg per day of diet cholesterol. Keep cholesterol 180 and below (chart inside front cover).

- Add 6 glasses of purified/distilled water daily to your diet. It's the best diuretic for a healthy heart. (Chlorinated/fluoridated water destroys vitamin E in the body.)

- Herbs for Blood Cleansing & Normalizing: Burdock Root, Sarsaparilla, Chaparral, Ginger & Licorice Root, Alfalfa, Red Clover, Green Tea, Dandelion, Sea Greens, Yellow Dock Root, Hawthorn Berry, Chlorella and Barley Grass.

  Super foods for heart therapy are Aloe Vera Juice & Gel, herbs, royal jelly, bee pollen and Siberian Ginseng.

Superfoods are foods found in nature. They are low in calories and high in nutrients. They are superior sources of anti-oxidants and essential nutrients.

*Excerpts from *Healthy Healing* – By Linda Page • www.healthyhealing.com

Dr. Linda Page's Herb & Supplement Therapy*

- **In an emergency:** 1 tsp. cayenne powder in water or juice, or cayenne tincture (20 drops) in water, may help bring a person out of a heart attack; or take liquid Carnitine as directed. Also one-half dropperful Hawthorn extract every 15 minutes.

- **Tone the heart muscle:** CoQ10 with E Tocotrienols (helps lower cholesterol). Ascorbate or Ester C with bioflavonoids, up to 5,000mg daily. Evening Primrose Oil 1,000mg 4 times daily. Magnesium rich herbs: Motherwort, Parsley or Magnesium 800mg.

- **Improve blood flow:** Red Sage tea or Gingko Biloba extracts 2-3 times daily, Creatine 3,000mg daily.

- **Antioxidants strengthen cardiovascular system and keeps it clear:** Hawthorn & Grapeseed 100mg 3x daily.

- **Boost your thyroid to reduce heart disease risk:** Spirulina, liquid chlorophyll, 2 Tbsp dry sea greens daily.

- **Cardiotonics help the heart beat stronger and steadier:** CoQ10 60mg 3x daily, Carnitine 1,000mg daily, Cayenne-Ginger caps or garlic caps 6x daily, Siberian Ginseng caps 2,000mg or the tea 2 cups daily and wheat germ oil caps for tissue oxygen.

- **Phyto-estrogen heart protective herbs for women on menopause:** Ginkgo Biloba extract helps prevent ischemia-caused fibrillation. Vitex (chaste tree berry) Extract and Licorice Root Tea (delicious when fasting).

- **Heart disease preventives:** Folic Acid – B6 -100mg & B12 - 2,500mcg, helps keep down homocysteine levels.

- **Reduce blood stickiness to prevent heart attack:** Bromelain 1,500mg regularly increases fibrinolysis (also Braggzyme helps, page 212 & 256), Chromium picolinate, Omega-3 fish or flax oil 3x daily.

- **To cleanse the arteries:** Vitamin E 800 IUs, Carnitine 1,000mg and Lysine and Arginine 2,000mg of each.

- **To help flush out infectious bacteria trapped in the blocked lymph glands and blood vessels:** Echinacea and Goldenseal extract in combination.

222

Dr. Linda Page's Lifestyle Support Therapy*

- Bite down on tip of little finger to help stop a heart attack.
- Apply hot compresses and massage chest to ease heart attack.
- Take alternate hot /cold showers to increase circulation.
- Smoking constricts the arteries and can cause your blood pressure to skyrocket. Researchers estimate that 150,000 heart disease deaths could be prevented each year if Americans just quit smoking! Quit smoking now! (pg. 75)
- Do mild regular daily exercise (preferably brisk walking). Do deep breathing exercises daily for more body oxygen to stimulate brain and to stay youthful with activity.
- Periodontal disease increases the chance of a heart attack by 2.7 times. Add CoQ10 – 100mg to your daily health program, good for teeth, gums and your heart!
- Add relaxation and a good daily laugh to your life. Also positive mental out-look does wonders for stress.

Dr. Linda Page's Heart Rehabilitation Program

This program is designed for those who have survived a heart attack or major heart surgery. Beginning and sticking to a new lifestyle that changes everything about the way you eat, exercise and handle stress, is a challenge. The following program is a blueprint you can use with confidence. It addresses main preventative needs – keeping your arteries clear and your blood slippery – goals that can be achieved through healthy diet and exercise.

- Reduce saturated fats to 10% of your diet; less if possible. Limit polyunsaturated oils to 10%. Add mono-unsaturates (olive oil, avocados, nuts and seeds). Add Essential Fatty Acids (fish, flax oil, etc.) Olive oil boosts healthy HDL-cholesterol levels and helps remove fats from blood. Bragg's Cold-Pressed Organic Extra Virgin Olive Oil is best, available health stores.

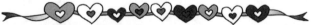

According to studies, periodontal disease can lead to serious complications for those with coronary heart disease. People with periodontal disease are twice as likely to develop cardiovascular disease. It's the bacteria from the mouth that enters the bloodstream and attaches to fatty proteins in blood vessels which may cause blood clots. While inflammation caused by periodontal disease may cause the arteries to harden. Brush your teeth and floss at lease twice daily and consult with your dentist.

*Excerpts from *Healthy Healing* – By Linda Page • *www.healthyhealing.com

- Eat potassium-rich foods for cardiotonic activity: spinach, chard, kale, broccoli, bananas, sea greens, molasses, apricots, cantaloupe, papayas, mushrooms, tomatoes and yams.

- Eat plenty of complex carbohydrates, such as broccoli, peas, whole grain breads, vegetable pastas, potatoes, sprouts, tofu and brown rice. Have a green salad every day.

- Have a couple of servings daily of foods like walnuts, ground flaxseed or flaxseed oil for essential omega-3 fatty acids.

- Eat magnesium-rich foods for heart regulation: tofu, wheat germ, oat or rice bran, broccoli, potatoes, lima beans, spinach, chard, bok choy and kale.

- Eat high-fiber foods for a clean system and alkalinity: whole grains, fruits and vegetables, legumes and herbs.

Almost all heart disease can be treated and prevented with improved nutrition. Refined, high fat, high calorie foods create heart problems. Natural, whole foods help relieve them! Full-fat dairy products like whole milk, ice cream and cheese are biggest dietary contributors to elevated LDL-cholesterol. Fried, salty, sugary foods, low-fiber, fatty and dairy foods, red meats, processed meats, tobacco and caffeine all contribute to clogged arteries, LDL bad cholesterol, high blood pressure and heart attacks!

Americans are in the highest risk category for heart disease. If you think conventional medicines will protect you, think again. Many experts think drug and surgical techniques to "protect" your heart are based on big bucks instead of health. Surgery alone cost Americans over $50 billion each year. Clearly, lives have been saved and extended, but drugs and surgery carry serious risks. New studies show that calcium channel blockers, the top selling blood pressure drugs, increase heart attack risk up to 60%. Many cholesterol-lowering statin drugs can cause serious liver toxicity, stomach distress and vision impairment. They also deplete CoQ10, an essential Coenzyme that strengthens the heart, by up to 50%.*

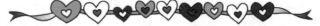

Herbs for Circulatory Stimulation: *Dandelion, Alfalfa, Sea Greens, Yellow Dock Root, Chlorella, Hawthorn Berry, Marshmallow, Barley Grass, Barberry Bark* Crystal Star Herbs available Health Food Stores or visit: www.HealthyHealing.com

Vitamin B12 is in sea greens, seaweed, soy foods, nutritional yeast, cereals and super greens like chlorella, spirulina and barley grass. If these foods are not in your vegetarian diet, it's vital to take vitamin B12, B6 and Folic Acid.

*Excerpts from *Healthy Healing* – By Linda Page • *www.healthyhealing.com*

Dr. Sinatra's Healthy Heart Program*

Dr. Sinatra strongly believes that the more efficient your body's cells are at creating and burning energy, the better your overall health will be. This is especially true of the heart, which uses more energy than any other organ in the body.

Dr. Sinatra's Top 12 Tips for a Healthy Heart

1. **Get on the modified healthy Mediterranean Diet.** I recommend this diet because it offers a combination of healthy fats, moderate protein and fewer carbohydrates – the optimal recipe for heart health. This diet is also rich in alpha-linolenic acid and omega-3 oils, which help prevent blood clotting, reduce blood pressure and prevent cholesterol buildup (see more on this diet page 226).

2. **Raise your fitness level.** I can't think of another lifestyle modification with such immediate and long-lasting benefits for your health and well-being. Even simple exercises strengthen your heart and circulatory system, build stamina and improve your state of mind! The best exercise is the one you will stick with. Walking and dancing are both great and enjoyable. Remember you don't have to work up a sweat or push yourself until you're out of breath.

   I wholeheartedly endorse weight-lifting to your exercise regimen to promote a healthy heart and bones. Not only does strength training increase endurance, it can promote healthy blood pressure and improve cholesterol levels and enhance your sense of well-being.

3. **Reduce your stress.** There are many effective stress-reduction techniques, such as: yoga, massage, prayer, visualization, deep breathing exercises, positive affirmations, listening to classical music and meditating or sitting quietly for 15 minutes a day.

225

Dancing Helps Your Heart: *A recent study has found that dancing has same benefit for heart patients as working out at the gym. Hit the dance floor and help your heart said readersdigest.com. I love dancing. I've danced the Polka with Lawrence Welk on TV show, danced with Fred Astaire, Gene Kelly, Bob Hope and Arthur Murray said, "You dance like a feather, you're the same size as my wife Katherine."* – PB

*See more excerpts on web: drsinatra.com – *Heart Health Center*

Dr. Sinatra's Top 12 Heart Tips continued*

4. **Take a multi-vitamin** that includes carotenoids, flavonoids, vitamins C, E and B and selenium.

5. **Co-Q10 Ubiquinol** is another strong must. It's one of the best nutrients for promoting heart health.

6. **L-Carnitine**, a nutrient that helps preserve heart health. Take 500mg to 2 grams daily.

7. **Magnesium and Calcium** promote healthy blood pressure and help regulate heart health. Calcium, which as a synergistic relationship with magnesium, promotes healthy blood vessels. Take daily together 500mg of magnesium and 1,000mg of calcium.

8. **Fish oil** is one of the best sources of healthy fat around. You can eat cold-water fish like salmon and mackerel or take fish or flax oil at least twice a week and/or take a daily fish/flax oil supplement.

9. **Smoking: Stop it!** Research shows that smokers are twice as likely to have serious heart problems.

10. **L-Arginine**, an amino acid that improves blood flow to the heart. Take 2 to 4 grams 2 hours before bedtime.

11. **Nattokinase** is very effective in breaking down fibrin which in turn helps keep blood free-flowing (see Braggzyme page 212 for more info).

12. **Alcohol: Limit it!** One glass of organic red wine daily with dinner is fine, if desired, but hard alcohol is out!

Dr. Sinatra's Diet Has Many Benefits*

After a great deal of research, I've concluded that the best overall diet is the Modified, Mediterranean Diet. This diet can support and balance blood sugar and insulin levels, while giving you more energy and helps you find ideal weight or body mass. This diet consists of:

• **Whole grains, raw nuts, seeds, soybeans and legumes** are the basic foundation. These foods provide complex carbohydrates, fiber, protein, vitamins and minerals. Complex carbohydrates are the "slow burners" – they convert to glucose slowly, support stable blood sugar levels, and don't convert to fat as easily as refined carbohydrates.

*Excerpts from: drsinatra.com – *Heart Health Center*

I recommend 1-2 small servings of organic whole grains and 1-2 servings of legumes daily. In terms of soy, 2 servings daily. Finally, 2-3 servings of raw nuts and seeds daily.

• **Fruits** have lots of water, fiber, antioxidants and vitamins and minerals. So, fill up on a delicious healthy fruit bowl! I recommend 1-2 servings of organic fresh fruit daily.

• **Vegetables** make preparing a nutritious, delicious, inexpensive meal easy and healthy. There are many organic vegetables to choose from. They are full of healthy nutrients and fiber. Use vegetables liberally to make great raw finger snacks, sandwiches and side dishes. I recommend 3-5 servings of organic fresh vegetables daily.

• **High-quality fats** – include olives and olive oil, fatty fish, raw nuts, nut butters, flaxseed, soy and avocados. I recommend 5-6 servings of healthy fats and oils daily.

• **Fish and eggs** are both important components. Both contain protein and essential fatty acids (EFAs). The right fish has health-boosting benefits. I feel strongly that you should choose toxic-free, migratory cold-water, fatty fish over meat and poultry as often as possible. I recommend 2-3 servings of wild (not farm-raised) fish weekly. Free-range eggs supply essential antioxidants. I recommend 3-6 a week.

• **Organic Dairy products** contain health-promoting calcium, protein, and vitamins B12 and D. I recommend no more than 2 servings per day and only organic!

• Eat in moderation 2-3 servings per week of **poultry** and just 1 serving per week or every other week of **beef or lamb** (be sure it is organic and hormone-free).

> **Here's Some Key Benefits of Mediterranean Diet:**
> Excerpts from: www.drsinatra.com – *Heart Health Center*

- High in healthy antioxidants
- High levels of healthy omega-3 fatty acids
- More fish, less beef and less dairy
- High in heart healthy olive oil
- Helps normalize your weight
- Higher energy levels and helps fight diseases
- Prevents blood clots, reduces blood pressure and helps prevent cholesterol build-up
- Can support more, even blood sugar levels

American Heart Association's Healthy Lifestyle

Excerpts from website: www.americanheart.org

Healthier lifestyle habits can help you reduce your risk for heart attack. Even simple small changes can make a big difference in your living a healthier, better life.

"Life's Simple 7" can help add years to your life:

1. Maintain a healthy weight
2. Eat a healthy diet
3. Engage in regular exercise
4. Don't Smoke
5. Manage blood pressure
6. Manage cholesterol
7. Keep blood sugar or glucose at healthy level

A healthy diet is one of your most powerful weapons in the fight against heart disease. Be sure to buy and eat plenty of organic fresh fruits and vegetables. Watch out for the saturated and/or partially hydrogenated fats hidden in bakery goods, casseroles, desserts and other foods. If desired have one serving of grilled or baked fish twice a week. Select more meat substitutes such as dried beans, peas, lentils and tofu and use them as entrees or in salads and soups. Raw nuts and seeds, are a good source of protein. Choose organic whole-grain, high-fiber breads.

Exercise more: swimming, cycling, jogging, skiing, aerobic dancing, walking or many other activities can help your heart. Whether it's included in a structured exercise program or part of your daily routine, all physical activity adds up to a healthier heart.

Your Daily Habits Form Your Future

Habits can be wrong or right, good or bad, healthy or unhealthy, rewarding or unrewarding. The right or wrong habits, decisions, actions, words or deeds . . . are up to you! Wisely choose your habits, as they can make or break your life! – Patricia Bragg, ND, PhD., Health Crusader

Many people say that cholesterol levels are not important. Caution! At Bragg we believe your blood cholesterol level is critical risk factor to determine your risk for heart disease. Dr. Dean Ornish and other leading health experts have demonstrated that by reducing blood cholesterol levels, you can not only prevent but even reverse heart disease. – Dr. John Westerdahl, Director Bragg Health Institute

Though no one can go back to the past and make a brand new start, you can start from right now and make a brand new healthier future! – Carl Bard

You are what you eat, drink, breathe, think, say and do! – Patricia Bragg

Chapter 22

Alternative Health Therapies And Massage Techniques

Try Them – They are Working Miracles for Millions!

Explore these wonderful natural methods of healing your body. Finally over 600 Medical Schools in the U.S. are teaching Healthy Alternative Therapies. Please check out the websites. Now seek and choose the best healing techniques for you:

ACUPUNCTURE/ACUPRESSURE **Acupuncture** directs and rechannels body energy by inserting hair-thin needles (*use only disposable needles*) at specific points on the body. It's used for pain, backaches, migraines and general health and body dysfunctions. Used in Asia for centuries, acupuncture is safe, virtually painless and has no side effects. **Acupressure** is based on the same principles and uses finger pressure and massage rather than needles. Websites offer info, check them out: *acupuncturetoday.com* or *acupressure.com*

CHIROPRACTIC Chiropractic was founded in Davenport, Iowa in 1885 by Daniel David Palmer. There are now many schools in the U.S., and graduates are joining Health Practitioners in all nations of the world to share healing techniques. Chiropractic is popular and the largest U.S. healing profession benefitting literally millions! Treatment involves soft tissue, spinal and body adjustment to free the nervous system of interferences with normal body function. Its concern is the functional integrity of the musculoskeletal system. In addition to manual methods, chiropractors use physical therapy modalities, exercise, health and nutritional guidance. Web: *chiroweb.com*

F. MATHIUS ALEXANDER TECHNIQUE These lessons help end improper use of neuromuscular system and bring body posture back into balance. Eliminates psycho-physical interferences, helps release long-held tension, and aids in re-establishing muscle tone. Web: *alexandertechnique.com*

FELDENKRAIS METHOD Dr. Moshe Feldenkrais founded this in the late 1940s. This Method leads to improved posture and helps create ease and more efficiency of body movement. This Method is a great stress removal. Web: *feldenkrais.com*

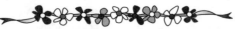

Physical Therapy & Massage helps promote healing & helps with respiratory, nervous disorders, asthma, emphysema, etc. It helps relieve pain, improve blood flow, helps correct posture & promotes health. – Dr. Linda Page, Author of *Healthy Healing*

Alternative Health Therapies & Massage Techniques

HOMEOPATHY In the 1800's, Dr. Samuel Hahnemann developed homeopathy. Patients are treated with "micro" doses of remedies found in nature to trigger the body's own defenses. This homeopathic principle is a safe and nontoxic remedy and is the #1 alternative therapy in Europe and Britain because it is inexpensive, seldom has any side effects, and usually brings fast results. Web: *www.homeopathic.org*

NATUROPATHY Brought to America by Dr. Benedict Lust, M.D., this treatment uses diet, herbs, homeopathy, fasting, exercise, hydrotherapy, manipulation and sunlight. (Dr. Paul C. Bragg graduated from Dr. Lust's first School of Naturopathy in the U.S. Now 6 schools) Practitioners work with your body to restore health naturally. They reject surgery and drugs except as a last resort. Web: *www.naturopathic.org*

OSTEOPATHY The first School of Osteopathy was founded in 1892 by Dr. Andrew Taylor Still, M.D. There are now 15 U.S. colleges. Treatment involves soft tissue, spinal and body adjustments that free the nervous system from interferences that can cause illness. Healing by adjustment also includes good nutrition, physical therapies, proper breathing and good posture. Dr. Still's premise: if the body structure is altered or abnormal, then proper body function is altered and can cause pain and illness. Web: *www.osteopathic.org*

REFLEXOLOGY OR ZONE THERAPY Founded by Eunice Ingham, author of *Stories The Feet Can Tell*, inspired by a Bragg Health Crusade when she was 17. Reflexology helps the body and organs by removing crystalline deposits from reflex areas (nerve endings) of feet and hands through deep pressure massage. Primitive reflexology originated in China and Egypt and Native American Indians and Kenyans self-practiced it for centuries. Reflexology activates the body's flow of healing and energy by dislodging deposits. Visit Eunice Ingham and nephew Dwight Byer's web: *www.reflexology-usa.net*

SKIN BRUSHING daily is wonderful for circulation, toning, cleansing and healing. Use a dry vegetable brush (never nylon) and brush lightly. Helps purify lymph so it's able to detoxify your blood and tissues. Removes old skin cells, uric acid crystals and toxic wastes that come up through skin's pores. Use loofah sponge for variety in shower or tub.

Alternative Health Therapies & Massage Techniques

REIKI A Japanese form of massage that means "Universal Life Energy." The Reiki Massage helps the body to detoxify, then re-balance and heal itself. Discovered in the ancient Sutra manuscripts by Dr. Mikso Usui in 1822. Web: *www.reiki.org*

ROLFING Developed by Ida Rolf in the 1930's in the U.S. Rolfing is also called structural processing and postural release, or structural dynamics. It is based on the concept that distortions (accidents, injuries, falls, etc.) and the effects of gravity on the body cause upsets and long-term stress in the body. Rolfing helps to achieve balance and improved body posture. Methods involve the use of stretching, gentle deep tissue massage and relaxation techniques to loosen old injuries, break bad movement and posture patterns. Web: *rolf.org*

TRAGERING Founded by Dr. Milton Trager M.D., who was inspired at age 18 by Paul C. Bragg to become a doctor. It is a mind-body learning method that involves gentle shaking and rocking, allowing the body to let go, releasing tensions and lengthening the muscles for more body peace and health. Tragering can do miracle healing where needed in the body frame, muscles and the entire body. Web: *trager.com*

231

WATER THERAPY Soothing detox shower: apply Bragg Olive Oil to skin, alternate hot and cold water, every 2-3 minutes. Massage body while under hot, filtered spray. Garden hose massage is great in summer or anytime. Hot detox soak bath (diabetics use warm water) 20 minutes with cup of Epsom salts or apple cider vinegar. This soak helps pull out the toxins by creating an artificial fever cleanse.Web: *holisticonline.com/hydrotherapy.htm*

MASSAGE & AROMATHERAPY works two ways: the essence (aroma) relaxes, as does healing massages. Essential oils are extracted from flowers, leaves, roots, seeds and barks. These are usually massaged into the skin, inhaled or used in a bath for their ability to relax, soothe and heal. The oils, used for centuries to treat numerous ailments, are revitalizing and energizing for the body and mind. Example: Tiger balm, MSM, echinacea and arnica help relieve muscle aches. (Avoid skin creams and lotions with mineral oil – it clogs the skin's pores.) Use these natural oils for the skin: almond, apricot kernel, avocado, and I use Bragg Organic Olive Oil and mix with aromatic essential oils: rosemary, lavender, rose, jasmine, sandalwood or lemon-balm, etc. – 6 oz. oil and 4 drops of an essential oil. Web: *naha.org*

Alternative Health Therapies & Massage Techniques

MASSAGE – SELF Paul C. Bragg often said, "You can be your own best massage therapist, even if you have only one good hand." Near-miraculous health improvements have been achieved by victims of accidents or strokes in bringing life back to afflicted parts of their own bodies by self-massage and even vibrators. Treatments can be day or night, almost continual. Self-massage also helps achieve relaxation at day's end. Families and friends can learn and exchange massages; it's a wonderful sharing experience. Remember, babies love and thrive with their daily massages, start from birth. Family pets also love their soothing, healing touch of massages. Web: *coolnurse.com/massage.htm*

MASSAGE – SHIATSU Japanese form of health massage that applies pressure from the fingers, hands, elbows and even knees along the same points as acupuncture. Shiatsu has been used in Asia for centuries to relieve pain, common ills, muscle stress and to aid lymphatic circulation. Web: *shiatsu.org*

MASSAGE – SPORTS An important health support system for professional and amateur athletes. Sports massage improves circulation and mobility to injured tissue, enables athletes to recover more rapidly from myofascial injury, reduces muscle soreness and chronic strain patterns. Soft tissues are freed of trigger points and adhesions, thus contributing to improvement of peak neuro-muscular functioning and athletic performance.

MASSAGE – SWEDISH One of the oldest and the most popular and widely used massage techniques. This deep body massage soothes and promotes healthy circulation and is a great way to loosen and relax tight muscles before and after exercise. Web: *massageden.com/swedish-massage.shtml*

232

Author's Comments: We have personally sampled many of these Alternative Therapies. It's estimated that soon America's health care costs will leap over $2 trillion. It's more important than ever to be responsible for our own health! This includes seeking holistic health practitioners who are dedicated to keeping us well by inspiring us to practice prevention! These Alternative Healing Therapies are also popular and getting results: aroma, Ayurvedic, biofeedback, color, guided imagery, herbs, music, meditation, magnets, saunas, tai chi, chi gong, Pilates, Rebounder, yoga, etc. Explore them and be open to improving your earthly temple for a healthy, happier, longer life. **Seek & find the best for your body, mind & soul. – Patricia Bragg, ND, PhD.**

Morning Resolve To Start Your Day

I will this day live a simple, sincere and serene life; repelling promptly every thought of impurity, discontent, anxiety, discouragement and fear. I will cultivate health, cheerfulness, happiness, charity and the love of brotherhood; exercising economy in expenditure, generosity in giving, carefulness in conversation and diligence in appointed service. I pledge fidelity to every trust and a childlike faith in God. In particular, I will be faithful in those habits of prayer, study, work, nutrition, physical exercise, deep breathing and good posture. I shall fast for a 24 hour period each week, eat only healthy foods and get sufficient sleep each night. I will make every effort to improve myself physically, mentally, emotionally and spiritually every day.

Morning Prayer used by Patricia Bragg and her father, Paul C. Bragg

Dear Friend, I wish above all things that thou may prosper and be in health even as the soul prospers. – 3 John 2

WE THANK THEE

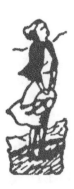

For flowers that bloom about our feet;
    For song of bird and hum of bee;
For all things fair we hear or see,
    Father in heaven we thank Thee!
For blue of stream and blue of sky;
    For pleasant shade of branches high;
For fragrant air and cooling breeze;
    For beauty of the blooming trees;
Father in heaven we thank Thee!
    For mother love and father care,
For brothers strong and sisters fair;
    For love at home and here each day;
For guidance lest we go astray,
    Father in heaven we thank Thee!
For this new morning with its light;
    For rest and shelter of the night;
For health and food, for love and friends;
    For every thing His goodness sends,
Father in heaven we thank Thee!

    – Ralph Waldo Emerson

233

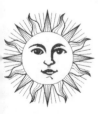

Count your blessings one by one and you will see what the Lord has done! I give thanks each day for all the miracle blessings I receive daily. – Patricia Bragg, ND, PhD.

A Personal Message to Our Students
The Body Self-Cleans & Self-Heals When Given A Chance

It is our sincere desire that each one of our readers and students attain this precious super health and enjoy freedom from all nagging, tormenting human ailments. After studying this healthy heart program, you know that most physical problems arise from an unhealthy lifestyle that creates toxins throughout the body. Many of these trouble hot spots are years old and are mainly concentrated in the intestines, colon and organs.

We have taught you that there is no special diet for any one special ailment! The Bragg Healthy Lifestyle promotes cleansing through the eating of more organic raw fruits and vegetables combined with regular fasting. It is only through progressive cleansing that the human *cesspool* can be banished! We have told you that you will go through healing crises from time to time. During these cleansing times you might have weakness and might become discouraged! This is the time you must have great strength and faith! It is during these crises, when you feel the worst, that you are doing the greatest amount of deep detox cleansing. This is why weaklings, and people without will-power and intestinal fortitude fail to follow this perfect Bragg Heathy Lifestyle System of Cleansing, Fasting and Rejuvenation! Please be strong!

Weaklings want a cure that requires no effort on their part. Mother Nature and your body do not work that way! The average unfortunate sick person thinks of the Lord as a kind and forgiving Father who will allow them to enter the Garden of Eden effortlessly and unpunished for any violation of His and Mother Nature's Laws.

You can create your own Garden of Eden anywhere you live, regardless of climate! You can reach a stage of health and youthfulness that you never thought was possible! You can feel ageless where your chronological age actually stands still and pathological age will make you younger! When your body is free of deadly toxic material you will reach the physical, mental, emotional and spiritual state that will give you happiness and it will add more youthful, active, joyous years to your life!

Earn Your Bragging Rights
Live The Bragg Healthy Lifestyle
To Attain Supreme Physical, Mental, Emotional and Spiritual Health!

With your new awareness, understanding and sincere commitment of how to live The Bragg Healthy Lifestyle – you can now live a longer, healthier life to 120 years! *(Gen. 6:3)*

God bless you and your family and may He give you the strength, the courage and the patience to win your battle to re-enter the Healthy Garden of Eden while you are still living here on Earth with more years to enjoy it all!

With Blessings of Health, Peace, Joy and Love,

Paul and *Patricia*

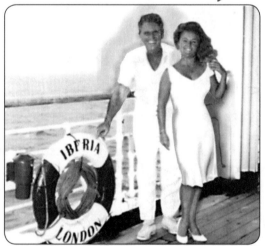

Health Crusaders Paul C. Bragg and daughter Patricia traveled the world spreading health, inspiring millions to renew and revitalize their health.
– 3 John 2
– Genesis 6:3

235

The Bragg books are written to inspire and guide you to health, fitness and longevity. Remember, the book you don't read won't help. So please reread Bragg Books and live The Bragg Healthy Lifestyle to enjoy a healthy fulfilled life!

I never suspected that I would have to learn how to live – that there were specific disciplines and ways of seeing the world that I had to master before I could awaken to a simple, healthy, happy, uncomplicated life.
– Dan Millman, Author of *The Way of the Peaceful Warrior* • www.danmillman.com
A Bragg fan and admirer since his Stanford University coaching days.

A truly good book teaches me better than to just read it,
I must soon lay it down and commence living in its wisdom.
What I began by reading, I must finish by acting! – Henry David Thoreau

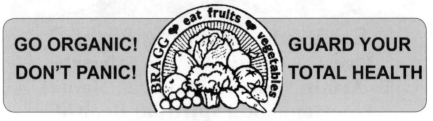

GO ORGANIC!
DON'T PANIC!

GUARD YOUR
TOTAL HEALTH

FROM THE AUTHORS

This book was written for You! It can be your passport to a healthy, long, vital life. We in the Alternative Health Therapies join hands in one common objective – promoting a high standard of health for everyone. Healthy Nutrition points the way – which is Mother Nature and God's Way. This book teaches you how to work with them, not against them! Health Doctors, Therapists Nurses, Teachers and Caregivers are becoming more dedicated than ever before to keeping their patients healthy and fit. This book was written to emphasize the great needed importance of healthy lifestyle living for health and longevity, close to Mother Nature and God.

Statements in this book are scientific health findings, known facts of physiology and biological therapeutics. Paul C. Bragg practiced natural methods of living for over 80 years with highly beneficial results, knowing that they were safe and of great value. His daughter Patricia lectured and co-authored Bragg Health Books with him and continues carrying on Bragg Health Crusades and Bragg Institute.

Paul C. Bragg and daughter Patricia express their opinions solely as Public Health Educators and Health Crusaders. They offer no cure for disease. Only the body has the ability to cure a person. Experts may disagree with some of the statements made in this book. However, such statements are considered to be factual, based on the long-time experience of dedicated pioneer health crusaders Paul C. Bragg and Patricia Bragg. If you suspect you have a medical problem, please always seek qualified health care professionals to help you make the healthiest, wisest and best-informed choices!

Count your blessings daily while you do your 30 to 45 minute brisk walks and exercises with these affirmations – health! strength! youth! vitality! peace! laughter! humility! understanding! forgiveness! joy! and love for eternity! and soon all these qualities will come flooding and bouncing into your life. With blessings of super health, peace and love to you, our dear friends – our readers. – Patricia Bragg, Health Crusader

Oxygen is the main nutrient of the body. When we improve our oxygen intake, we enhance our immune system and the body's ability to detoxify and stay healthy for a long life. – Dr. Michael Schachter, Columbia University

If I were to name the three most precious resources of life, I would say books, friends and nature; and the greatest of these, at least the most constant and always at hand is Mother Nature and God. – John Burroughs

236

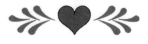

When you sell a man a book you don't just sell him paper, ink and glue, you sell him a whole new life! There's heaven and earth in a real book, and the main purpose of books is to trap the mind into its own thinking and action. – Christopher Morley

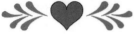 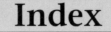 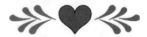

Follow the steps of the godly instead, and stay on the right path, for good men enjoy life to the full. – Proverbs 2:20-21

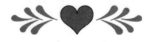

Index

Touch is a primal need, as necessary as food, clothing or shelter. Michelangelo knew this when he painted God extending a hand toward Adam on the ceiling of the Sistine Chapel, he chose touch to depict the gift of life. – George H. Colt

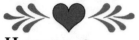 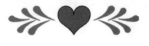

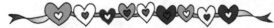

Wherever there is a human being there is an opportunity for kindness. – Seneca

When you can think of yesterday without regret, and of tomorrow without fear, then you are on the road to peaceful success.

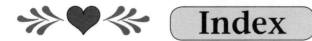 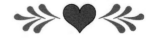
Love, kindness and compassion are necessities, not luxuries . . . without them humanity cannot survive. – The Dalai Lama, Bragg Liquid Aminos Fan

241

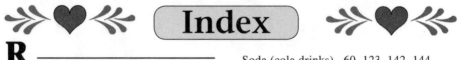

Index

Love is the sun shining in us to sparkle our lives! – Patricia Bragg, ND, PhD.

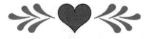 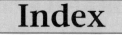 # Index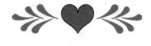

HAVE AN APPLE HEALTHY LIFE!

THE MIRACLES OF APPLE CIDER VINEGAR FOR A STRONGER, LONGER, HEALTHIER LIFE

> **The old adage is true:**
> *"An apple a day keeps the doctor away."*

- Helps promote a youthful skin and vibrant healthy body
- Helps remove artery plaque and body toxins
- Helps fight germs, viruses, bacteria and mold naturally
- Helps retard old age onset in humans, pets and farm animals
- Helps regulate calcium metabolism
- Helps keep blood the right consistency
- Helps regulate women's menstruation, relieves PMS, and UTI
- Helps normalize urine pH, relieving frequent urge to urinate
- Helps digestion, assimilation and balances the pH
- Helps relieve sore throats, laryngitis and throat tickles and cleans out throat and gum toxins
- Helps protect against food poisoning and brings relief if you get it
- Helps detox the body so sinus, asthma and flu sufferers can breathe easier and more normally
- Helps banish acne, athlete's foot, soothes burns, sunburns
- Helps prevent itching scalp, baldness, dry hair and helps banish dandruff, rashes, and shingles
- Helps fight arthritis and helps remove crystals and toxins from joints, tissues, organs and entire body
- Helps control and normalize body weight

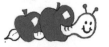

– Paul C. Bragg, Health Crusader,
Originator of Health Stores

Our sincere blessings to you, **dear friends,** who make our lives so worthwhile and fulfilled by reading our teachings on natural living as our Creator laid down for us to follow. He wants us to follow the simple path of natural living. This is what we teach in our books and health crusades worldwide. Our prayers reach out to you and your loved ones for the best in health and happiness. We must follow the laws He has laid down for us, so we can reap this precious health physically, mentally, emotionally and spiritually!

HAVE AN APPLE HEALTHY LIFE!

With Love,

244

Bragg's Organic Raw Apple Cider Vinegar with the "Mother" is the #1 food I recommend to maintain the body's vital acid-alkaline balance, plus digestion.
– Gabriel Cousens, M.D., Author, Conscious Eating

BRAGG "HOW-TO, SELF-HEALTH" BOOKS
Authored by America's First Family of Health
Live Longer – Healthier – Stronger Self-Improvement Library

Qty.	BRAGG Book Titles Health Science ISBN: 978- 0-87790	Price	$ Total
	10 BRAGG Book Offer – Get Healthy, Live Longer Special – plus Free SH .....only 89.00		
	(Please see next 2 pages for book descriptions)		
_____	**Apple Cider Vinegar Miracle Health System** – *(over 8 million in print)* 9.95		
_____	**Back Fitness Program** – For Pain-Free, Strong, Healthy Back 9.95		
_____	**Bragg Healthy Lifestyle** – **Vital Living to 120** (formerly Toxicless Diet)................... 9.95		
_____	**Build Powerful Nerve Force** – Increase Energy, Eliminate Fatigue, Stress, Anger, Anxiety 11.95		
_____	**Build Strong Healthy Feet** – Banish Aches & Pains, Dr Scholl said "it's the best"......... 8.95		
_____	**Healthy Heart** – Keep Your Heart & Cardiovascular Healthy & Fit at any age................ 11.95		
_____	**The Miracle of Fasting** – Bragg Bible of Health, Physical Rejuvenation & Longevity .. 11.95		
_____	**Super Power Breathing** – for Super Energy, Longevity, & Heal Asthma, Allergies 11.95		
_____	**Water, The Shocking Truth** – That Can Save Your Life - Learn safest water to drink 8.95		
_____	**Vegetarian Health Recipes** – 700 Delicious, Nutritious, Healthy Recipes 13.95		
	BRAGG DVD – Enjoy BRAGG History, Lectures, Exercise Class, etc......................only 7.95		

| TOTAL COPIES | Books also available as E-books - see bragg.com
Due to printing/paper costs, prices subject to change without notice. | **TOTAL BOOKS** $ | |

Please Specify: ☐ Check   ☐ Money Order   ☐ Credit Card

Books Only: CA Residents add 8.75% tax

(S&H) Shipping & Handling

Charge To: ➤   ☐ Visa   ☐ Master Card   ☐ Discover

Month   Year
|
Card Expires

VISA   MasterCard   DISCOVER

CVV #:

Credit Card Number

Signature

(USA Funds Only)
TOTAL BOOKS $

| USA Shipping | Please add $5 first book,
$1 each additional book
USA retail book orders over $50 add $7 only |
| International Shipping | Canada add $11 for first book.
$1.50 each additional book
All other Int'l. orders add $13.
$1.50 each additional book |

CREDIT CARD ORDERS ONLY
CALL **(800) 446-1990**
8 am-4 pm PST • Mon.-Fri.
OR FAX **(805) 968-1001**

Business office calls **(805) 968-1020**. We accept MasterCard, Discover or VISA phone orders. Please prepare order using this order form. It will speed your call and serve as your order record.
Hours: 8 am to 4 pm Pacific Time, Monday thru Friday.
• Visit our Web: www.bragg.com • e-mail: bragg@bragg.com

See & Order Bragg "Bound" Books, E-Books, & Products on www.bragg.com
Mail to: **HEALTH SCIENCE, Box 7, Santa Barbara, CA 93102 USA**
Please Print or Type – Be sure to give street & house number to facilitate delivery.

BOF 111

Name
Address   Apt. No.
City   State   Zip
( )
Phone   e-mail

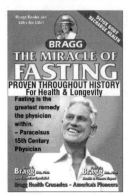
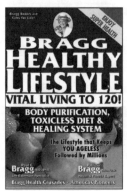
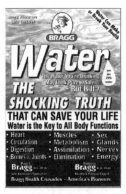
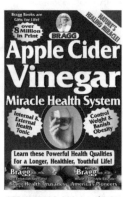
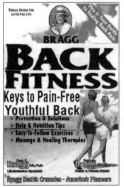
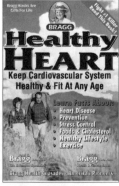

246

BRAGG HEALTH BOOKS ARE GIFTS FOR LIFE

Gen. 6:3 · 3 John 2

– Jack LaLanne, Bragg follower since 15 years old

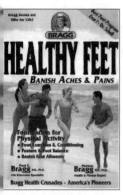

Learn how to banish aches & pains. Read about Reflexology, Acupressure and much more. Almost all of us are born with perfect feet. It's the abuse millions give their feet that makes them cry as they limp through life - "my aching feet are killing me!" Read this book!

The Bragg Foot Program is the best. I thank Bragg Books and their wisdom for my long, active, healthy life.
– Dr. Scholl,
Famous Foot Doctor

0-87790-077-9 – \$8.95

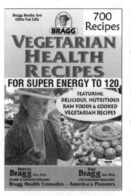

Enjoy the worlds finest health recipes for super health and high energy that you and your family will love. Over 700 Healthy Recipes for Health, Super Energy and Longevity. 326 pages filled with delicious raw and cooked foods, vegan and vegetarian recipes.

This book shows how to eat right with nutritious recipes to maintain the body's health and fitness.
– Henry Hoegerman, M.D.

978-0-87790-027-6 – \$13.95

Millions of healthy, happy followers have learned to control and increase their Vital Nerve Force Energy - the Bragg Healthy Way. Here's Prevention and Health Maintenance all in one book.

I have my life back after many years of chronic fatigue, fibromyalgia and clinical depression. I give thanks to The Bragg Health Books.
– Marilyn Mason

978-0-87790-093-1 – \$11.95

Breathing deeply, fully and completely energizes, calms, fills you with peace and keeps you youthful. Learn Bragg Breathing Exercises for more go-power and Super Health!

Thanks to Paul Bragg and Bragg Books, my years of asthma were cured in only one month with The Bragg Super Breathing and Bragg Healthy Lifestyle Living!
– Paul Wenner
Gardenburger Creator

978-0-87790-120-4 – \$11.95

"I thank Paul Bragg and the Bragg Healthy Lifestyle for my healthy, long, active life." I love Bragg Books and Health Products."
– Jack LaLanne, Bragg follower since 15 years old

I have followed "The Bragg Healthy Lifestyle for years and it teaches you to take control of your health and build a healthy future."
– Mark Victor Hansen, Co-Producer *Chicken Soup for the Soul* Series

"Thanks to Bragg Books for my conversion to the healthy way."
– James F. Balch, M.D.
Co-Author of – *Prescription for Nutritional Healing*

"Bragg Books have been a blessing to our family and the TBN family of loyal viewers"
– Evangelist Dwight Thompson - *Co-Host TBN "Praise The Lord"*

If Bragg Books are unavailable in your area you may order: on-line at: www.bragg.com or see Bragg book list. Bragg Book Special: All 10 books for only \$89 Postpaid.

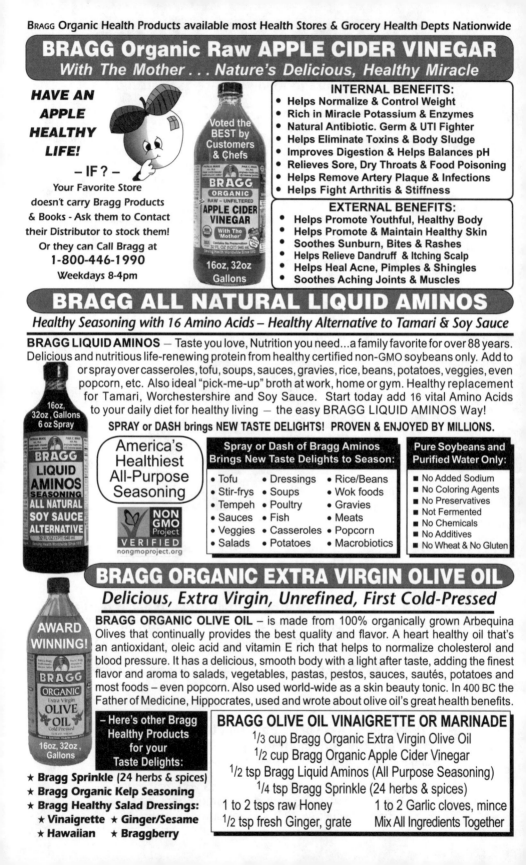

BRAGG ORGANIC APPLE CIDER VINEGAR

SIZE	PRICE		UPS SHIPPING & HANDLING For USA	$ Amount
16 oz.	$ 3.29	each	S/H – Please add $9. for 1st bottle and $1.50 each additional bottle	.
16 oz.	$ 36.00	Special Case /12	S/H Cost by Time Zone: CA $12. PST/MST $14. CST $22. EST $25	.
32 oz.	$ 5.29	each	S/H – Please add $10. for 1st bottle – $2. each additional bottle	.
32 oz.	$ 58.00	Special Case /12	S/H Cost by Time Zone: CA $17. PST/MST $20. CST $35. EST $38	.
1 gal.	$ 16.49	each	S/H – 1st bottle: CA $10. PST/MST $10. CST $13. EST $15 – $6. each add'l bottle	.
1 gal.	$ 57.00	Special Case /4	S/H Cost by Time Zone: CA $17. PST/MST $20. CST $34. EST $37	.

BRAGG Vinegar is a food and not taxable

BRAGG VINEGAR	$.
(S&H) Shipping & Handling	.
TOTAL	$.

BRAGG LIQUID AMINOS

SIZE	PRICE		UPS SHIPPING & HANDLING For USA	$ Amount
6 oz.	$ 3.59	each	S/H – Please add $9. for 1st 3 bottles – $1.50 each additional bottle	.
6 oz.	$ 78.00	Special Case /24	S/H Cost by Time Zone: CA $10. PST/MST $11. CST $17. EST $19	.
16 oz.	$ 4.69	each	S/H – Please add $9. for 1st bottle – $1.50 each additional bottle	.
16 oz.	$ 51.00	Special Case /12	S/H Cost by Time Zone: CA $12. PST/MST $14. CST $22. EST $25	.
32 oz.	$ 7.69	each	S/H – Please add $9. for 1st bottle and $2. each additional bottle	.
32 oz.	$ 84.00	Special Case /12	S/H Cost by Time Zone: CA $17. PST/MST $20. CST $35. EST $38	.
1 gal.	$ 28.39	each	S/H – 1st bottle: CA $10. PST/MST $10. CST $13. EST $15 – $6. each add'l bottle	.
1 gal.	$ 99.00	Special Case /4	S/H Cost by Time Zone: CA $17. PST/MST $20. CST $34. EST $37	.

BRAGG Aminos & Olive Oil are foods and not taxable

BRAGG AMINOS	$.
(S&H) Shipping & Handling	.
TOTAL	$.

BRAGG ORGANIC OLIVE OIL

SIZE	PRICE		UPS SHIPPING & HANDLING For USA	$ Amount
16 oz.	$ 10.99	each	S/H – Please add $9. for 1st bottle – $1.50 each additional bottle	.
16 oz.	$ 120.00	Special Case /12	S/H Cost by Time Zone: CA $12. PST/MST $14. CST $22. EST $25	.
32 oz.	$ 17.89	each	S/H – Please add $10. for 1st bottle and $2. each additional bottle	.
32 oz.	$ 196.00	Special Case /12	S/H Cost by Time Zone: CA $17. PST/MST $20. CST $35. EST $38	.
1 gal.	$ 62.69	each	S/H – 1st bottle: CA $10. PST/MST $10. CST $13. EST $15 – $6. each add'l bottle	.
1 gal.	$ 219.00	Special Case /4	S/H Cost by Time Zone: CA $17. PST/MST $20. CST $34. EST $37	.

Please Specify: ☐ Check ☐ Money Order ☐ Cash
Charge to: ☐ Visa ☐ Master Card ☐ Discover

Credit Card Number: _____

Card Expires: _____ / _____ month / year

BRAGG OLIVE OIL	$.
(S&H) Shipping & Handling	.
TOTAL	$.

VISA

MasterCard

DISCOVER

Signature: _____

Business office calls (805) 968-1020. We accept MasterCard, Discover & VISA phone orders. Please prepare order using order form. It speeds your call and serves as order record. Hours: 8 to 4 pm Pacific Time, Monday thru Friday.

• Visit our Web: www.bragg.com • e-mail: bragg @ bragg.com

CREDIT CARD ORDERS
CALL **(800) 446-1990**
8 am-4 pm PST • Mon.-Fri.
OR FAX **(805) 968-1001**

Mail to: **HEALTH SCIENCE, Box 7, Santa Barbara, CA 93102 USA** BOF 111
Please Print or Type – Be sure to give street & house number to facilitate delivery.

Name _____

Address _____ Apt. No. _____

City _____ State _____ Zip _____

Phone ( ) _____ e-mail _____

Bragg Health Products available most Health Stores & Grocery Health Depts Nationwide

Bragg Organic Products available Health Stores & Grocery Health Depts Nationwide

BRAGG HEALTHY SALAD DRESSINGS

ORGANIC HEALTHY VINAIGRETTE

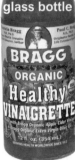

This Bragg Healthy Organic Vinaigrette Dressing makes a salad special with its tasty, tangy flavor. A zesty blend of Bragg Organic Extra Virgin Olive Oil, Bragg Organic Apple Cider Vinegar, Bragg Liquid Aminos, garlic, and onion, raw honey and delicious organic herbs. This unique taste brings you a healthy dressing with the Bragg's best tradition of healthy eating and healthy living.

12 oz glass bottle

NEW

BRAGGBERRY Dressing & Marinade

Brings new taste treats, with Blueberries, Raspberries, Acai, Goji and Grape. Low-fat and natural antioxidants. All of the best of Bragg's tradition of healthy eating and living.

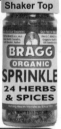

12 oz glass bottle

12 oz glass bottle

Made with Organic GINGER & SESAME

This Bragg Healthy Dressing is based on the delicious flavors of our famous Bragg Liquid Aminos and ginger's sweet and tangy taste. Great on salads and veggies, brings you the best of Bragg tradition of healthy eating and living.

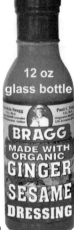

12 oz glass bottle

BRAGG HAWAIIAN Dressing & Marinade

Brings Taste of Aloha to salads, veggies, stir-frys and other healthy foods. Unlock Hawaiian secret flavors you will love with Bragg Natural Delicious and Tasty Hawaiian Dressing and Marinade.

America's Healthiest All-Purpose Seasonings

BRAGG SPRINKLE
ORGANIC 24 HERBS & SPICES

This old favorite is now available again. Bragg Sprinkle was created in 1931 by Paul C. Bragg, Health Pioneer & Originator Health Food Stores. Organic Sprinkle adds new healthy, delicious flavors to most recipes & meals. It's salt-free with no additives, preservatives or fillers.

Shaker Top

BRAGG ORGANIC KELP SEASONING

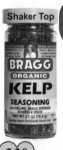

Shaker Top

This original Organic Kelp Seasoning made from sun-dried Organic Pacific Ocean Sea Kelp, combined with 24 all natural herbs and spices. It's a healthy, delicious seasoning for almost all recipes and meals and is specially suited for low-sodium diets.

NEW

BRAGG
Delicious
Nutritional
Yeast Seasoning

Nutritionally designed to help meet nutritional needs of vegetarians, vegans and anyone wanting a good source of B12, B-Complex Vitamins. It's "cheese-like" flavor makes it a delicious, healthy seasoning.

Shaker Top

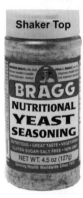

- Gluten-Free • Non-GMO
- No Salt • No Sugar • No Dairy
- No Artificial Colors & Preservatives
  - No Brewery Products
  - No Candida Albicans
- Vegetarian & Kosher Certified

250 *You are what you eat, drink, breathe, think, say & do.* – Patricia Bragg, ND, PhD.

BRAGG SPRINKLE – 24 Herbs & Spices Seasoning

SIZE	PRICE	UPS SHIPPING & HANDLING For USA	$	Amount
1.5 oz.	$ 4.69 each	S/H – Please add $9. for 1st 3 bottles and $1. each additional bottle		.
1.5 oz.	$ 51.00 Special Case /12	S/H Cost by Time Zone: CA$9. PST/MST $9. CST $10. EST $12.		.
BRAGG Sprinkle Seasoning is a food and not taxable		BRAGG SPRINKLE	$	.
		(S&H) Shipping & Handling		.
		TOTAL	$	.

BRAGG ORGANIC SEA KELP

2.7 oz.	$ 4.69 each	S/H – Please add $9. for 1st 3 bottles and $1. each additional bottle		.
2.7 oz.	$ 51.00 Special Case /12	S/H Cost by Time Zone: CA$9. PST/MST $9. CST $10. EST $12.		.
BRAGG Kelp Seasoning is a food and not taxable		BRAGG KELP	$	.
		(S&H) Shipping & Handling		.
		TOTAL	$	.

BRAGG NUTRITIONAL YEAST

4.5 oz.	$ 6.29 each	S/H – Please add $9. for 1st 3 bottles and $1. each additional bottle		.
4.5 oz.	$ 69.00 Special Case /12	S/H Cost by Time Zone: CA$9. PST/MST $9. CST $10. EST $12.		.
BRAGG Nutritional Yeast Seasoning is a food and not taxable		BRAGG YEAST	$	.
		(S&H) Shipping & Handling		.
		TOTAL	$	.

BRAGG SALAD DRESSINGS

✳ BRAGG GINGER & SESAME SALAD DRESSING

12 oz.	$ 5.49 each	S/H – Please add $9. for 1st bottle and $1.25 each additional bottle		.
12 oz.	$ 60.00 Special Case /12	S/H Cost by Time Zone: CA$11. PST/MST $12. CST $19. EST $22		.

✳ BRAGG ORGANIC VINAIGRETTE SALAD DRESSING

12 oz.	$ 5.49 each	S/H – Please add $9. for 1st bottle and $1.25 each additional bottle		.
12 oz.	$ 60.00 Special Case /12	S/H Cost by Time Zone: CA$11. PST/MST $12. CST $19. EST $22		.

✳ BRAGG BRAGGBERRY DRESSING & MARINADE

12 oz.	$ 5.49 each	S/H – Please add $9. for 1st bottle and $1.25 each additional bottle		.
12 oz.	$ 60.00 Special Case /12	S/H Cost by Time Zone: CA$11. PST/MST $12. CST $19. EST $22		.

✳ BRAGG HAWAIIAN DRESSING & MARINADE

12 oz.	$ 5.49 each	S/H – Please add $9. for 1st bottle and $1.25 each additional bottle		.
12 oz.	$ 60.00 Special Case /12	S/H Cost by Time Zone: CA$11. PST/MST $12. CST $19. EST $22		.
BRAGG Salad Dressings/Marinades are foods and not taxable		BRAGG SALAD DRESSINGS	$	.
		(S&H) Shipping & Handling		.
		TOTAL	$	.

Payment Method:

☐ Check   ☐ Money Order   ☐ Cash   **Charge To:** ☐ Visa   ☐ Master Card   ☐ Discover

Credit Card
Number:_____

Card
Expires:_____ / _____
month / year

Signature:_____

Business office calls (805) 968-1020. We accept MasterCard, Discover & VISA phone orders. Please prepare order using order form. It speeds your call and serves as order record. Hours: 8 to 4 pm Pacific Time, Monday thru Friday. • Visit our Web: www.bragg.com • e-mail: bragg @ bragg.com

CREDIT CARD ORDERS
CALL **(800) 446-1990**
8 am - 4 pm PST • Mon.- Fri.
OR FAX **(805) 968-1001**

Mail to: **HEALTH SCIENCE, Box 7, Santa Barbara, CA 93102 USA**   BOF 111
Please Print or Type – Be sure to give street & house number to facilitate delivery.

Name _____

Address _____   Apt. No. _____

City _____   State _____   Zip _____

( ) _____   _____
Phone   e-mail

Bragg Products available most Health Stores & Grocery Health Depts Nationwide

BRAGG ORGANIC APPLE CIDER VINEGAR DRINKS

ENERGY BOOSTERS

ORGANIC THIRST QUENCHERS

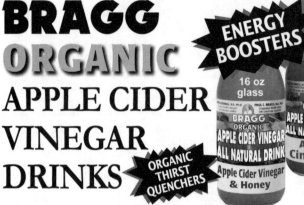

16 oz glass

16 oz glass

16 oz glass

16 oz glass

Apple Cider Vinegar & Honey

Apple - Cinnamon

Ginger Spice

Grape Acai

Enjoy Healthy Goodness and Taste of BRAGG Organic Apple Cider Vinegar in Energizing, Refreshing Health Drinks.

Delicious, ideal pick-me-up for home, work, gym or sports. Perfect taken as healthy thirst quencher & energy booster.

- Based on Paul & Patricia Bragg's Original Recipe
- Natural Goodness of Bragg Organic Apple Cider Vinegar
- Sweetened with Organic Honey or Organic Natural Stevia
- Great-Tasting, Healthy Refreshing Drinks
- Great for a Quick Energy Boost
- Convenient Pre-mixed Drinks
  (two 8-oz. servings per bottle)
- Certified Organic and Kosher Certified
- Try Drinks Today! Your Body and You will Love them!

Discover the Power of BRAGG Organic Apple Cider Vinegar.

USDA ORGANIC

All Flavors Contain two 8 oz. servings

Made with "World Famous" Bragg Organic Apple Cider Vinegar & Organic Raw Honey

4 Choices:
- Apple Cider Vinegar & Honey
- Apple-Cinnamon • Ginger Spice
- Concord Grape-Acai

In 400 BC Hippocrates, the Father of Medicine, used Apple Cider Vinegar for its amazing natural detox cleansing, healing, and energizing qualities. Hippocrates prescribed ACV mixed with honey for its health properties.

BRAGGZYME ®

Powerful Systemic Enzymes for Active Lifestyle and Heart Support

Dr. Paul C. Bragg, the first to introduce enzyme supplements in 1931. Now Bragg Health Science is proud to introduce most advanced systemic enzyme supplement, Braggzyme – that contains powerful 500mg Complex Formula (Nattokinase, Serrapeptase, Bromelain, Papain, Protease and Lipase).

BRAGGZYME™ Superior Systemic Enzymes provide nutritional and cardiovascular support you need to help maintain a normal inflammatory response and maintain safe fibrin levels for a healthy cardiovascular system.* Braggzyme contains no animal derivatives, no artificial flavors, no artificial coloring, no yeast and no wheat.

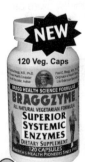

NEW

120 Veg. Caps

BRAGGZYME
ALL NATURAL VEGETARIAN FORMULA
SUPERIOR SYSTEMIC ENZYMES
DIETARY SUPPLEMENT
120 CAPSULES

- Enzyme support for back, joints, muscles, tendons and immune system.*
- Boost energy levels – infuses life-giving oxygen to every cell in body.*
- Nutritional support to help maintain a normal inflammatory response.*
- Helps eliminate dangerous fibrin levels for a healthier blood flow.*
- 4,500 Fibrinolytic Units (FU) per cap to help normalize healthy fibrin levels.*
- Helps keep your hands and feet and entire body warm.*
- Helps keep your memory and brain more sharp.*
- 100% Safe, All Natural Vegetarian Formula in Veg. cap.

252

*These statements have not been evaluated by the Food & Drug Administration. This product is not intended to diagnose, treat, cure, or prevent any disease.

BRAGG ORGANIC APPLE CIDER VINEGAR DRINKS

FLAVORS	SIZE	PRICE	QTY	CASE PRICE	QTY	$	Amount
Original Apple Cider Vinegar & Honey - 16 oz		$2.19		$24.00			.
ACV with Ginger - Spice - 16 oz		$2.19		$24.00			.
ACV with Apple - Cinnamon - 16 oz		$2.19		$24.00			.
ACV with Concord Grape - Acai - 16 oz		$2.19		$24.00			.

**BRAGG ORGANIC APPLE CIDER VINEGAR DRINKS
are Foods and are not taxable**

BRAGG VINEGAR DRINK $ ___ .

(S&H) Shipping & Handling

SHIPPING CHART FOR ACV DRINKS ↙

number of bottles	CA	PST/MST	CST	EST
1-2 bottles	$8.00	$8.00	$9.00	$12.00
3-4 bottles	$8.00	$9.00	$11.00	$13.00
5-6 bottles	$9.00	$9.00	$13.00	$15.00
7-12 bottles	$11.00	$13.00	$21.00	$24.00
Special Case/12	$11.00	$13.00	$21.00	$24.00

TOTAL $ ___ .

**Please call around to
Health & Grocery Stores
first, because many are
now selling Bragg Products.**

BRAGGZYME – Systemic Enzymes

SIZE	PRICE	UPS SHIPPING & HANDLING For USA	$	Amount
120 cap	$ 43.95 each	S/H – Please add $9. for 1st 3 bottles and $1. each additional bottle		.
120 cap	$ 483.00 Special Case /12	S/H Cost by Time Zone: CA $9. PST/MST $10. CST $11. EST $12.		.

on Braggzyme CA Residents only pay tax

**for BRAGGZYME only
CA Residents add 8.75% TAX** $ ___ .

(S&H) Shipping & Handling

TOTAL $ ___ .

Payment Method:

☐ Check   ☐ Money Order   ☐ Cash

Charge To: ☐ Visa   ☐ Master Card   ☐ Discover

Credit Card
Number: _____

Card
Expires: ___ / ___
month / year

Signature: _____

VISA

MasterCard

DISCOVER

Business office calls (805) 968-1020
We accept MasterCard, Discover & VISA
Phone orders please prepare order using order forms,
as it speeds up your call and serves as your order record.
Hours: 8 to 4 pm Pacific Time, Monday thru Friday.
• Visit Web: www.bragg.com • e-mail: bragg @ bragg.com

CREDIT CARD ORDERS
CALL **(800) 446-1990**
8 am - 4 pm PST • Mon.-Fri.
OR FAX **(805) 968-1001**

Mail to: **HEALTH SCIENCE, Box 7, Santa Barbara, CA 93102 USA**
Please Print or Type – Be sure to give street & house number to facilitate delivery.   BOF 111

Name

Address   Apt. No.

City   State   Zip

( )
Phone   e-mail

Bragg Products available most Health Stores & Grocery Health Depts Nationwide

Send for Free Health Bulletins

Patricia wants to keep in touch with you, your relatives and friends about the latest Health, Nutrition and Longevity Discoveries. Please enclose one stamp for each USA name listed or visit *www.bragg.com* and sign up for literature.

With Blessings of Health, Peace and Thanks

Patricia

Please make copy, then print clearly and mail to:

BRAGG HEALTH CRUSADES, Box 7, Santa Barbara, CA 93102

Name
_____

Address _____ Apt. No. _____

City _____ State _____ Zip _____

Phone ( ) e-mail _____

- -

Name
_____

Address _____ Apt. No. _____

City _____ State _____ Zip _____

Phone ( ) e-mail _____

- -

Name
_____

Address _____ Apt. No. _____

City _____ State _____ Zip _____

Phone ( ) e-mail _____

- -

Name
_____

Address _____ Apt. No. _____

City _____ State _____ Zip _____

Phone ( ) e-mail _____

- -

Name
_____

Address _____ Apt. No. _____

City _____ State _____ Zip _____

Phone ( ) e-mail _____

Bragg Health Crusades spreading health worldwide since 1912

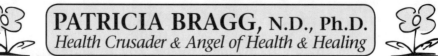

PATRICIA BRAGG, N.D., Ph.D.
Health Crusader & Angel of Health & Healing

Author, Lecturer, Nutritionist, Health & Lifestyle Educator to World Leaders, Hollywood Stars, Singers, Athletes, etc. & Millions

Patricia is a 100% health crusader with a lifetime dedication passion like her father, Paul C. Bragg, world renowned health authority. Patricia has won international fame on her own. She conducts Bragg Health & Fitness Seminars & Lectures for Conventions & Schools, Women's, Men's, Youth & Church Groups world-wide. She promotes Bragg Healthy Lifestyle Living & "How-To, Self-Health" Books on Radio & TV Talk Shows throughout the English-speaking world. Consultants to Presidents & Royalty, to Stars of Stage, Screen & TV & to Champion Athletes, Patricia & her father co-authored The Bragg Health Library of Instructive, Inspiring Books that promote a healthier lifestyle, for a long, healthy, happy life.

Patricia herself is the symbol of health, perpetual youthfulness & natural femininity, radiant & super energy. She is a living & sparkling example of her & her father's healthy lifestyle precepts & this she loves sharing world-wide.

A fifth-generation Californian on her mother's side, Patricia was reared by The Bragg Natural Health Method from infancy. In school, she not only excelled in athletics, she won honors for her studies & counseling. She is an accomplished musician & dancer, tennis player & mountain climber. Patricia is a popular gifted Health Teacher, a dynamic personality & perfect Talk Show Guest on Radio & TV Shows where she regularly spreads the simple, easy-to-follow Bragg Healthy Lifestyle for everyone of all ages. Patricia's been on the covers of many magazines as her health message is needed & well received by millions.

Man's body is his vehicle through life, his earthly temple & the Creator wants us filled with joy & health for a long, fulfilled life. The Bragg Crusades of Health & Fitness (3 John 2) has carried her around the world over 30 times – spreading physical, emotional, mental & spiritual health & joy. Health is our birthright & Patricia teaches how to prevent the destruction of our health from man-made wrong lifestyle habits of living.

Patricia's been a Health Consultant to American Presidents, British Royalty, to Champion Triathletes *(She wrote 600 page Tri-Health Fitness Manual)*, Betty Cuthbert, Australia's "Golden Girl" (16 world records & 4 Olympic track gold medals), & New Zealand's Olympic Track & Triathlete Star, Allison Roe. Among those who follow her advice are some of Hollywood's top Stars from Clint Eastwood to ever-youthful singing group – The Beach Boys, Singing Stars of Metropolitan Opera & top Ballet Stars, etc. Patricia's message is of world-wide appeal & well received by people of all ages, nationalities & walks-of-life. Those who follow The Bragg Healthy Lifestyle & attend The Bragg Crusades world-wide are living testimonials . . . like ageless, super athlete, Jack LaLanne, who at age 15 went from sickness to Total Fitness & Health!

Patricia inspires you to Renew, Rejuvenate and Revitalize your Life with "The Bragg Healthy Lifestyle" Books and Health Crusades worldwide. Millions have benefitted from these life-changing events with a longer, healthier and happier life! She loves to share with your community, organization, church groups, etc. Also, she is a perfect radio and TV talk show guest to spread the message of healthy lifestyle living. See and hear Patricia on the web: bragg.com For radio interview & lecture requests write or e-mail: **patricia@bragg.com**
BRAGG HEALTH CRUSADES, BOX 7, SANTA BARBARA, CA 93102, USA